The Least Among Thee

TO BE A CHRISTIAN – TO BE A PHYSICIAN

Jan van Eys, MD, PhD

Clinical Professor of Pediatrics, Emeritus
Vanderbilt University, School of Medicine
Nashville, Tennessee

ISBN: 1484003012
ISBN-13: 9781484003015
Library of Congress Control Number: 2013908099
CreateSpace Independent Publishing Platform North Charleston, SC

The AIN Ministry Invites You to a
Conference for Physicians

POINT AND COUNTERPOINT.....

Physician and Theologian in Dialogue

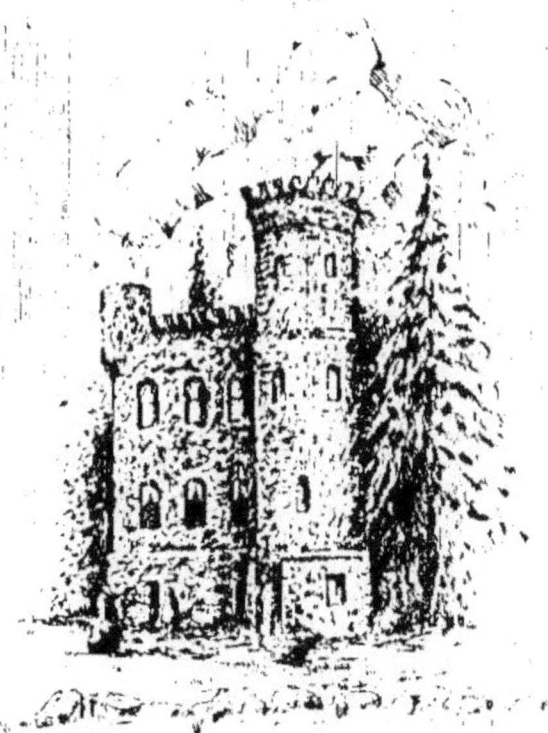

LEADER: Jan Van Eys, Ph.D., M.D.

SPONSOR: Westminster Presbyterian Church
          47 Jefferson S. E.
          Grand Rapids, MI 49503
          (616-456-1456)

DATES: September 18, 19, 20, 1981

          Approved for CME credit

To my late wife, who taught me how to communicate love,
and to my children, who make me grateful to be a father.

ACKNOWLEDGMENT

Barbara Reschke, at the University of Texas M.D. Anderson Cancer Center, edited the first version of this book with loving care and great concern. Authors are deeply indebted to their editors. Editors are the first ones who must try to understand what was meant the way it was written. That is not always easy.

PREFACE

All of us struggle with the absolute at one time or another. If we do not willingly join the struggle, sooner or later it engages us. We may find ourselves in the lines of Robert Frost:

> I am too absent-spirited to count.
> The loneliness includes me unawares.[1]

Physicians struggle all the time – they have engaged the absolute by answering their calling. They must answer all the questions that confront them daily in human suffering and misery, in death and survival.

Many such physicians profess to be Christians. If we pose as axioms that we are Christian, that we believe in our profession and in the way we would like to exercise our skills, where do we then go? Ought that set of axioms not guide us to the answers to our questions? We feel as we did in our geometry classes when we did not truly know whether our answers were correct until our teacher checked them. But the degree with which we were at ease when we handed them in was a reasonable clue to the grade we were to get.

There is surprisingly little literature on what it means to be a physician. There is rather too much about the patient-doctor relationship, and far too much about medical expertise and the limits of medical authority. There is a reasonable amount about the development of medicine from the priesthood, but most, if not all, of this literature is a reflection in the general. The Christian encounter is always in the specific, even if our expression of love may require the expression of general concerns.

This book deals with what it means to be a physician, and it attempts to answer in Christian symbolism and realities. So much more could have been said: the work could have been turned into a scholarly tome, but that would have diluted the expression of experience. Much of what is said is generally applicable. In our society, physicians are the most frequently consulted professionals in time of stress. Their lives are, however, only a concentrated version of the lives of all humans. There is a far greater residuum of the priesthood of the physician than we normally acknowledge.

The book is based on a workshop, "*Point and Counterpoint: Physician and Theologian in Dialogue*," which took place in 1981. Many of the quotes were from the time the workshop was held or shortly thereafter. Medical science has progressed enormously since then, especially in the application of molecular biology and genetics to therapeutics. Simultaneously the business of medicine became more prominent. But those developments have only sharpened the emphasis on the mechanics of medicine away from care. Nothing has changed in the argument offered in this book.

TABLE OF CONTENTS

INTRODUCTION

In 1981 my wife and I were invited by the Westminster Presbyterian Church in Grand Rapids, Michigan to participate in a retreat workshop on being a Christian and a physician. The workshop was called "*Point and Counterpoint: Physician and Theologian in Dialogue.*" I was asked to be the leader. Physicians and their spouses were invited as couples. The workshop was held at *the Castle*, a venerable and rustic hotel on the grounds of a long-established vacation-home community on the shore of Lake Michigan.[1]

The church was a most generous host, and we expected that. But we were little prepared for the experience that weekend turned out to be. The setting of the Castle was unique in itself, and ideally suited for the mood in which the weekend was spent. I was told that *The Wizard of Oz* was written at Castle Park. While it was far from Kansas, we found the same searching mood to be present, and the realization that our courage must come from our own resources. We were not prepared for the intensity of dialogue and the openness of sharing of concerns, but the atmosphere, the new friends, and the pervasive feeling of genuine Christian commitment generated a flow of ideas that became a beautiful whole. The experience will never be duplicated for us. Yet memories fade so fast. There is so much more to remember than just a mood and a feeling. There was a realization that it is possible to formulate what it is to be a Christian and a physician in such a way that one becomes a Christian physician.

Not only did we find the heart to acknowledge it and the brain to express it, but all of us there also found the courage within ourselves to share it.

I wrote a recollection of that weekend and the thoughts we worked through. It was neither a diary nor a transcription; rather, it was the consequence of reflection on what happened there in Michigan. It was not a treatise either: it was written shortly after the event.

What spurred the writing then was my experience as a member of the taskforce on Science, Health, and Human Values of the Advisory Council on Church and Society of the Presbyterian Church. A discussion between scientists, physicians, and theologians in which I had the privilege of participating made it abundantly clear that true dialogue is not possible until one understands the concepts behind the words one uses. When I, as a physician, wanted to use the words that theologians taught me, I first had to master and appropriate the concepts. It is one thing to learn the language out of a phrase book and therewith meet a pragmatic necessity. It is another to truly learn a language so that ideas, rather than things, can be expressed. Once I began to understand theological language I began to realize the radical and self-negating concepts Christianity forces upon us. If we don't realize that, our words will sound at worst hollow, and at best amusing, to the tolerant listener.

This book is, therefore, the product of both an experience and a perceived need. It was also the product of a long and happy marriage. Wives were invited to the Castle because they share with their husbands the agony of being a physician. By accident and not by design, no female physicians were present. My wife, who was a professional in oral deaf education, and I, a pediatric oncologist, had supported each other in our moments of doubt and despair and rejoiced for each other in our moments of certainty. The ideas expressed in this book did not just emerge on that weekend in the Fall – they were all there, already shaped in understanding dialogue between my wife and me. However, they did become a unified whole during that one remarkable experience in Michigan.

Then the book was set aside for over two decades. It seemed I had to live out what I tried to say. Theory and practice are two very different touchstones. But once a theory is formulated it is just fluff unless tested.

Medicine must be lived out. Patients may have had all kinds of thoughts about what they must do when ill and what rules physicians ought to follow. However, when patients are really sick, when the reality of possible death faces them, they have to learn to trust. They have to choose a physician whom they can trust to help when self-help is beyond their power. They have to learn to have faith in a God who will help whatever may happen.

Even physicians who become patients learn that lesson. Lewis Thomas, who served as president and later as director of the Memorial Sloan Kettering Cancer Center, was a celebrated commentator on modern medicine and biological sciences. When he had an emergency pace maker installed because of severe cardiac arrhythmias, he should have been the ideal subject for informed consent. But he wrote about his surprise:

> I do not want to know about my new technology. I do not even want to have reasons for needing it fully explained to me. As long as it works, and it does indeed, I prefer to be as mystified by it as I can. This is a surprise. I would have thought that as a reasonably intelligent doctor-patient, I would be filled with intelligent, penetrating questions, insisting on comprehending each step in the procedure, making my own decisions, even calling the shots. Not a bit of it. I turn out to be the kind of patient who doesn't want to have things explained only to have things looked after by real professionals. Just before I left the hospital, the cardiologist brought me a manila envelope filled with reprints, brochures, [and] the manufacturer's instructions for physicians listing all indications, warnings, and the things that might go wrong. I have the envelope somewhere, on a closet shelf I think, unexamined. I haven't, to be honest, the faintest idea how a pacemaker works, and I have even less curiosity.[2]

Lewis Thomas learned that all his theoretical preaching about the boundary between patient and physician was but theory. He had to trust the professional.

Some years later my wife was admitted to an intensive care unit for chest pain and a slow heart rate. She had a near cardiac arrest, fortunately after admission. An emergency pacemaker was inserted, followed shortly thereafter by a permanent one. She was grateful for the extra years granted her by God through medicine. I had to learn to entrust her care to my colleagues.

The caring physicians must live out those encounters too. They are the instruments of God through which life must be extended. They must learn to be trustworthy in order to be trusted. However, what implications does "being trustworthy" have? What does it mean to be an instrument of God?

The reflections in my first draft were not wrong. I would have made them again after such an encounter in the Castle. However, the next nearly twenty-five years were essential to finalizing the book. In that interval I continued to take care of children with cancer. I had to confront life-threatening illness where my skills or my mistakes might make a difference. I had to teach my trainees what it means to be a physician, technically, ethically, and spiritually. I had to struggle with care for the poor in a rich but aloof environment. I met many persons with greater experience and wisdom than I had or ever will have. All those experiences leavened the reflections.

We retired. Then my wife died of cancer, the very disease to which I dedicated my professional life in order to learn how to conquer it. This gave the final perspective on faith and service. It was good the workshop was held when I was younger. Ideas were expressed with greater conviction and discussed with greater vigor than would have been done after mellowing by experience and loss, by failure and success.

Here then is the final record of a remarkable week and the impact it has made on a rich life as a physician, teacher, spouse, and father.

CHAPTER I

The Christian and the Medical Profession

The need to have faith in what one does is obvious. The ability to have faith in what one does, requires the ability to believe that what one does is good. That is an extremely difficult posture to maintain. Physicians cannot continually extract justification out of themselves. They must find a certainty within themselves.

Physicians are healers. They must have a position of faith that allows them to survive the ontological onslaught that the continuous confrontation with the sick presents.

Christianity is a foundation that can support a faith that allows a doctor to be a faithful healer without being overwhelmed by the patients' illnesses. Once patients have trust and faith in what the physician offers, all the ontological meaning that the patient attributes to being ill, becomes part of the healing target.[1]

To be a Christian is, in itself, a commitment that requires defining. However, it is not my purpose to make Christianity itself the object of scrutiny. It is assumed that those physicians who are in dialogue with me through this book are, indeed, Christians as much as they are physicians. The question is not how a physician can be a Christian but how a Christian can be a physician in the best tradition of healing and caring.

In the final analysis, a Christian is defined as one who believes in Jesus Christ. Many confessions have attempted to pin down that assertion. Church dogma traditionally has professed that faith in creeds. It will, therefore, be understood as axiomatic that a profession of faith, such as is embodied in the Apostles Creed, is accepted. I grew up in a culture that uses a language other than English to communicate the Word. Our common source for this most generally used Creed is worded in Latin:

Credo in Deum Patrem Omnipotentem, Creator Coeli et Terrae.

Et in Iesum Christum, Filium eius unicum, Dominum nostrum,
qui conceptus est de Spiritu Sancto, natus ex Maria Virgine;
passus sub Pontio Pilato, crucifixus, mortuus, et sepultus;
descendit ad inferna, tertia die resurrexit a mortuis, ascendit ad coelos,
sedet ad dextram Dei Patris omnipotentis, inde venturus est judicare vivos
et mortuos.

Credo in Spiritum Sanctum, sanctam ecclesiam catholicam,
sanctorum communionem, remissioneum peccatorum, carnis resurrec-
tionem; vitam aeternam.

Amen.

Even though it has been translated into many languages, often with selected omissions or redactions, the original Creed stands. We recite it in many churches in unison:

I believe in God, the Father Almighty, maker of Heaven and Earth.

And in Jesus Christ, His only begotten Son, our Lord, who was conceived by the Holy Spirit, born of the Virgin Mary, suffered under Pontius Pilate, was crucified, dead, and buried. He descended into Hell. The third day He rose again from the dead. He ascended into heaven and sits on the right hand of God, the Father Almighty. From there he shall come to judge the quick and the dead.

The Christian and the Medical Profession

I believe in the Holy Spirit, the holy catholic Church, the communion of the Saints, the forgiveness of sins, the resurrection of the body, and life everlasting.

Amen.

When we recite it, we must, at least on occasion mean it, if we do not want to live a sham. Just as it is necessary to have faith in one's profession to be a trustworthy physician, so it is necessary to believe in one's Creed to be a Christian. Of course, we all have our doubts at times. There are implications in the Creed that might keep one from approaching Christ. To quote Thielicke:

The fact is that I am not very happy about erecting the super-steep wall of the Apostle's Creed in our services of worship, nor about the many who are hungry and thirsty, the people for whom the promises of faith were intended but who suddenly grow faint and lapse into silence.

And yet there is one good thing about this steep wall: it prevents one from sliding by too easily and makes it impossible to keep on revolving in the circle of discussion.[2]

One must know medicine to be a physician; one must have a creed to be a Christian. Physicians constantly face challenging decisions, which they must and can make because at that moment they *know*. Whether that knowledge for decision comes from facts remembered, reading of textbooks and literature, or consultation is irrelevant. When we repeatedly are asked to reassert our Christianity, we can do so because we *believe*. Whether we have at that moment no debilitating doubt, whether we seek solace from the Bible, or whether we seek strength in prayer is irrelevant.

However, the mere statement *that* we believe is inadequate. Christianity as a belief offers a promise of help and redemption. The Almighty God and the mortal human will inevitably be in conflict. We will act out our

The Least Among Thee

Prometheus legend repeatedly when, as physicians, we challenge the course of the very nature of life. Christianity allows us then to seek forgiveness when we have taken on the burden of decision-making and when we *per force* have sinned because of that. When we recite, "I believe in Jesus Christ, His only begotten Son," we "step into the great center of the Christian Creed," to quote Karl Barth.[3]

That is the part that allows one to be a physician. To believe in Christ is not enough. To believe in redemption is a necessary component of our faith. To juxtapose and merge being a physician and being a Christian is possible only when we accept as axiom that we are both. Being a physician is difficult in itself, quite apart from the perceptions of that faith we have.

My personal experience as a physician has come from my practice as an Academic pediatric hematologist/oncologist. That practice may appear too extreme to serve as an example for all medicine. Extreme cases do indeed make bad law. However, extreme cases can also make the commonplace clearer. What will be said about caring for children with life-threatening diseases applies to care for all patients who seek our help.

In our Western world one specializes as much in Christianity as one does in medicine. In that arena, I speak from the experience of a Methodist who had a modern Calvinistic-Dutch Reformed upbringing. That makes me a trifle less specialized than in matters medical. However, no matter what subspecialty the person-to-person encounter between patient and doctor is a general one, as is the encounter of person to God.

Physicians in America, in modern times, are said to practice scientific medicine. That is, however, not synonymous with practicing medicine scientifically. Scientific medicine uses scientific discoveries to help design treatments for patients. Practicing medicine scientifically means that one uses the principles of scientific research in one's approach to developing the treatments. The former, as far as it goes, is a statement of fact. The latter is almost an accusation, even when the clinical trial is touted as the best approach to care. Not infrequently doctors almost believe that this accusation is a compliment.

"Scientific medicine" means only that the means we have at our disposal to treat are derived from facts and observations acquired through the scientific method. But science is never enough; there is far more to medicine. "To practice medicine scientifically," on the other hand, means to do clinical research. There is nothing inherently wrong with that whenever research is needed to obtain information in order to practice scientific medicine. However, patients do not understand that concept. Patients must trust their physicians to serve them best. Yet physicians have uncertainties about the basis of their calling and the means by which they must practice.[4]

Scientific medicine is frequently hailed as a major accomplishment of modern Western society. The impact of scientific medicine on understanding and thereby on preventing disease is enormous. General mortality patterns have changed. Causes of death have been identified. This has shortened the course of many diseases. Some historical scourges have become treatable or, even better, preventable. Even when not preventable yet, they have changed from plagues to inconveniences. It is, therefore, easy to assume that cures are modern medicine's triumphs. Cures, however, contribute only a small amount to the overall decline in mortality. Modern hygiene has prevented epidemics; application of epidemiological knowledge has contained disease outbreaks; nutritional knowledge has prevented crippling of children – the list is very long. However, its cure is not the reason that tuberculosis has declined. Antibiotics have not controlled typhoid fever; insulin has not solved diabetes; digitalis has not cut cardiovascular mortality; and cyclophosphamide is not going to solve cancer, nor is any new chemotherapeutic agent.

Those statements are statistical facts. Diseases decimate populations; the halting of a disease will have long-range impact on future generations. Such arguments, however, ignore the *patient* with cancer; they only address the *disease* cancer. In a war, the armies win but the soldier suffers; in modern medicine, science wins and the patient can become just a statistic. When I am well, I want the problem of cancer solved; when I have cancer, I want to be cured.

The tragedy of our age is that the promises for the future are thought to be the help of today. The accomplishments of science are interpreted as panaceas for us, here and now. Sometimes that does happen. At other times, the results of scientific medicine are not available, yet the relief of symptoms that does happen is interpreted as one more triumph of what medicine has to offer. But most of the times what is hailed as a breakthrough is no help for sufferers now. Where, then, is medicine when we really need it? Where is the cure for cancer? Medicine does not have an unequivocal answer; all it has to offer is a method for achieving the cure. The method is at best experimental therapy and at worst a vague hope and a promise.

It is no wonder that the promise of an easy cure attracts. The professionals of medicine only offer vague hopes; the testimony of fellow sufferers seems to hold out easy cures. The cures do not even need to be easy; they can be arduous, if only they promise success. Even if they only promise occasional success, they can still be selected over medical science. We usually contrast such choices as the lure of lore over science. For the outsider the choice appears obvious, but usually it is not. What is lore and what is science is not always clear. Much lore is steeped in tradition; much experimental therapy is unconventional by anyone's measure. Nor is it always a choice between lay and professional. There is lore among the professionals – more than we would like to admit. Physicians all have their shibboleths that may do little harm, but do not deserve the conviction with which they are dispensed. The extreme lore is quackery – and there are almost as many professional quacks as there are snake-oil dispensers.

The definition of what is lore and what is science shifts continuously. Folk medicine has given scientific medicine invaluable cures. There are relatively few drugs that medicine could not do without. Until recently digitalis was high on the list of such drugs. Digitalis was, in the form of foxglove leaves, a folk medicine to alleviate dropsy long before it became a mainstay of scientific cardiology. The story of licorice remains fascinating. Many patients with adrenal insufficiency in the Netherlands survived during World War II, even though hormone replacement therapy was unavailable. The reason could be traced to the national habit of eating salted licorice. That relationship, in turn, led to further understanding of the function of the adrenal glands and the mechanisms at work in hypertension. In cancer, the drug vincristine comes from the lowly periwinkle plant; cytosine arabinoside was found in the primitive sponge. It is, of course, the nature of scientific medicine to recognize such clues, to understand them, and to progress from there. It was not the discovery of penicillin that constituted the genius of the discoverer, but the recognition that the product of a mold, which contaminated bacterial cultures, was significant.

The medicine of the establishment is not always easy to take. We laugh at the description of seventeenth century medicine. Consider the treatment of King Charles II of England:

> As the first step in the treatment the king was bled to the extent of a pint from a vein in his right arm. Next his shoulder was cut into and the incised area was "cupped" to suck out an additional eight ounces of blood. After this homicidal onslaught the drugging began. An emetic and purgative was administered and soon after a second purgative. This was followed by an enema containing antimony, sacred bitters, rock salt, mallow leaves, violets, beetroot, chamomile flowers, fennel seed, cinnamon, cardamom seed, saphron, cochineal, and aloes. The enema was repeated in two hours and a purgative given. The king's head was shaved and a blister raised on his scalp. A sneezing powder of hellebore root was administered, and also a powder of cowslip flowers "to strengthen his brain." The cathartics were repeated at frequent intervals, and interspersed with a soothing drink composed of barley water, licorice, and sweet almond. Likewise, white wine, absinthe and anise were given, as also were extracts of thistle leaves, mint, rue and angelica. For external treatment a plaster of burgundy pitch and pigeon dung was applied to the king's feet. The bleeding and purging

continued, and to the medicaments were added melon seeds, manna, slippery elm, black cherry water, an extract of flowers of lime, lily-of-the-valley, peony, lavender, and dissolved pearls. Later came gentian root, nutmeg, quinine, and cloves. The king's condition did not improve; indeed it grew worse, and in the emergency forty drops of extract of human skull were administered to allay convulsions. A rallying dose of Raleigh's antidote was forced down the king's throat; this antidote contained an enormous number of herbs and animal extracts. Finally bezoar stone was given. Then says Scarburgh: "Alas! After an ill-fated night his serene majesty's strength seemed exhausted to such a degree that the whole assembly of physicians lost all hope and became despondent: still so as not to appear to fail doing their duty in any detail, they brought into play the most active cordial." As a sort of grand summary of this pharmaceutical debauch a mixture of Raleigh's antidote, pearl julep, and ammonia was forced down the throat of the dying king.[5]

A course of intensive chemotherapy could be described in the same way, and our children's children will laugh about it. To the child with cancer now, it is not the least bit funny. Yet, it is the best we have to offer, just as the king demanded treatment from the best medical brains of the day. We would say he was lucky if he had survived it; so is the person lucky who has completed a course of intensive chemotherapy and lives. Remember, many patients in heart failure were significantly improved by blood-letting. We now remove excess fluids with pills called diuretics, but the principle is no different. Not all folk medicine is foolish philosophy. Often valid observations strengthen therapeutic practices, just as we see cures from our chemotherapeutic regimens.

On what basis then does the patient choose between lore and science? Not the statistical likelihood that scientific medicine is superior. Statistics are for populations, not individual people. The answer is far more personal; it lies in the expectations of the patient and also in the faith of the providers of medical care in their product. The expectation of the patient is not the hope for a cure – that is too general and too obvious. Rather, the answer is determined by what a cure means to a patient. To ask for a cure is to express a need. The person, who fulfills that need, will sell the patient on the cure. A patient's needs are multiple and at many levels – except on an intellectual and reasoned level – and never just the removal of the disease.

To have cancer is to have pain, discomfort, and threat of death. It is being different from others; it is loneliness; loss of control over destiny; disfigurement. It is to be touched by the Almighty. But how that touch is felt, where the pressure is the heaviest, is very different for each patient. Relief of pain can be the immediate and overriding goal, to be sought at all cost, but by what a patient is further motivated is different for each. The fear of losing a self-image of physical integrity may make one teenager unable to face the recommendation for amputation. Another fears the self-disintegration that loss of control means, to such a degree that care must be manipulated to magnify the illusion of self-determination. There are so many sick persons out there that a purveyor of promises will always strike somebody as the bearer of miracles.

There is nothing wrong with supporting patients in whatever area they feel most threatened. When patients complain about the impersonality of modern medicine, they are almost always complaining about the lack of sensitivity toward their specific problem. It is quite feasible to remain attuned to the individual concerns each patient brings with his or her disease. Physicians, nurses, social workers and all others touching upon the patients' care can become friends who will support the patients in their needs. Humanizing medical care is a concern of the establishment as well as of patients and their families. Therefore, the needs of the patient, once recognized, should not be the overriding determinant in choosing between lore and science. Human needs can be met in either.

There is no doubt that modern medical institutions are impersonal. The more life-threatening the illness, the bigger and farther away from home the center usually is. The more specialized the center, the less the people there seem to understand the patient behind the illness. But the personnel is composed of persons too. Patients can find friends with whom they can share concerns. To ask the friendly family physician to care beyond his ken is to choose lore, not science; it is not necessary. To feel like a number is to expect the institution to assign a name, but the patient has a name already; to be treated as a person the patient has to behave like one. Even the most impersonal center is still only a small corner of the whole world. Friendship is possible and concerns can be voiced and heeded.

What makes a patient decide to choose between alternatives is not just the promise, not just the difficulty of achieving personal contact, but rather the faith that the system has in itself. A system that has no faith in itself will not attract new members; it will, in fact, not long endure. The choice between apparently easy cure and scientific medicine will tip toward easy cure if scientific medicine is unsure about itself. Even now, scientific medicine could easily have the strong upper hand. Negative anecdotes notwithstanding, the medical achievements have been so great that great expectations are justified. Patients can recognize that the so-called "easy cure" is really a failure, despite the positive anecdotes surrounding it. People will always choose the convinced prophet because of his apparent unquestioned calling, demonstrated by faith in himself.

The successful peddlers of quackery have faith in themselves. The more dishonest, the more likely that faith is. If the ultimate goal is easy money and if the product delivers, faith radiates because of the quack's certainty of the outcome. The suffering of the victim is of no consequence, not because the charlatan is necessarily hardened, but because it does not occur to him or her that the suffering is as serious as it really is. Whatever conscience they have is soothed by a variation on the theme that a freedom of choice is being offered.

There are, of course, deluding healers who have, themselves, a misplaced faith in their method. Many faith healers truly believe. Such people, when they discover their ineffectiveness, suffer the torments of hell that exceeds the combined physical and mental suffering that they leave in their wake. Adelle Davis died of cancer. When she was told that she had Multiple

The Christian and the Medical Profession

Myeloma, after so many years of promising health to all her followers, she was quoted as saying that she was "shocked ... fearful ... panicky ... I could not think straight." [6] However, she never lost faith: "I tell you this: I am trying some pretty unconventional things. Frankly, I'd be very surprised if I die of cancer. I'm eating better than ever." But she did die of cancer, leaving many frightened people who lost their easily understandable messiah.

Other prophets did lose their faith completely. Spas have flourished and vanished. Some shrines have attracted multitudes and are long forgotten. Miracles are claimed, verified, denounced, all to no avail. But the lack of success of shrines never contributed to their decline. Lack of healing showed lack of faith on the part of the ailing. Just as following doctor's orders is required to partake of medical help, so is faith required to partake of miracles. Lack of faith is, in a way, analogous to lack of compliance. What makes shrines falter is the inability of pilgrims to retain faith. The caretakers of the shrine, the peddlers of the remedy, all must be able to instill faith. Such faith is instilled by the faith the proponents of the cure have in themselves and their message.

There are signs of disillusionment with classical and scientific medicine. That means there is a problem within medicine itself and not that a stronger power lies within the alternatives. Modern medicine is not becoming less effective – quite the contrary. The tools of modern medicine are very powerful indeed. A good example is the solution of Legionnaire's disease that occurred in 1976: a new disease was recognized; its cause identified; the epidemiology defined; and treatment found. [7] The problem with modern medicine is entirely analogous to that of the religion behind the shrine. The god did not become less powerful; the ability to proclaim that power decreased.

Therefore, if a shift in mood and utilization of modern medicine is occurring, it means only one thing: a loss by the medical community of faith in itself and its approach. Not a disillusionment of the public, not a stronger siren song, but a wavering of physicians themselves as to whether what they are doing is really right.

The Least Among Thee

Modern scientific medicine is a process that hopes to achieve ultimate control of disease. But the system does not concede that the ultimate solution is around the corner. Rather, the process of getting there is what generates the power. For those diseases where cure is not yet known, the voice of scientific medicine says, "Experimental therapy is the best therapy." It does not say, "Experimental therapy is the best we have to offer," but rather "It is the best." The process of research has supplanted the goal. Research has become a way of care and no longer exclusively a means toward an end.

Many physicians do not understand any longer where experiment stops and standard therapy starts. Experiments have a way of failing. Each experiment has an *a priori* likelihood of significant advance, and that likelihood has been low; otherwise, progress would have been far faster. On the other hand, success has not been so infrequent that the experiments needed to be abandoned. Progress has been real and, in the course of human events, even rapid; though in the course of one patient's disease, slow. As experiment became a way of life and care, the faith that pulled patients toward participating was the sincere belief that the experimental way was indeed the optimal way of caring for the sick. There are many rewards in the mode of scientific medicine for physicians, from federal support through esteem through plaudits of peers.

But the faith is faltering. It is not really clear why. Fiscal austerity has decreased the positive financial reinforcement. Only in pediatrics have results been good enough to foster continued belief in the ultimate success of cancer cure. Debates about ethics place the decision of right and wrong about medical activities beyond the physician. Acknowledging the possibility of malpractice confuses experiment and care. Identity crises occur among paramedical personnel, from nurses through social workers to pharmacists. Probably the strongest factor in the decline of faith is that there is no common enemy to fight. There is no competing therapy that challenges certainties and thereby makes them more secure. Doctors of osteopathy are now recognized as "Doctors of medicine" in most states. Holistic medicine does not challenge, because it does not attack the principles, only the system. There is ennui in medicine that undermines the faith of the doctors. Medical school applicants are dropping; fellowships are not filled.

A collectively faltering faith cannot be restored. A single sinner can be restored to the fold, but prevailing doubt by the community destroys a denomination. If scientific medicine is the choice that offers the patient the best hope, an internal renewal is necessary to restore the faith of the doctors, not the faith of the patients. The greatest saints of the church are those who achieved church renewal, not those who converted the most heathens. Renewal implies the strengthening of the positive but also the discarding of the negative.

The first step in reasserting faith in medicine is a clarification of purpose. It is vital that research and standard care be clearly separated. It is vital that patients and parents be made partners with physicians in research, so that mutual trust becomes reestablished. Guidelines for research in children, and the concepts underlying it, must be completely acceptable and, what is more, accepted. Over the years this issue has been discussed extensively,[8] but a great deal of confusion remains in the minds of doctors and nurses and all others concerned. Our uncertainty generates uncertainty in the patient; the patient wonders if the doctors know what they are doing. When it is standard care, the answer is "yes." When it is a research project, the answer is "no." But doctors should know why they are doing the research and how it is to be done; that is the value of research. If the doctors are clear when they are researching, and the patient is clear what mode of care is offered, no uncertainties exist and faith in our care can be restored.

It is essential that doctors reestablish personal criteria about the appropriateness of care and research. Judgments on research made to accommodate institutional review boards (IRBs) are made too late.[9] To submit a research proposal should imply that there is a personal conviction that the research is necessary. The medical question to be answered must be valid, the science sound, and the patient risk, if any, acceptable. The research on therapy must first be ethically justified in the mind of the researcher.

The Least Among Thee

The IRB really only poses the question of whether the investigator plans to be honest with the patient. The motivation for research should be to solve the question itself, not to generate last-ditch therapy for the patient. That means that clarity of ethics and clarity about the boundary between research and care are strongly related. If last-ditch therapy is a by-product of the research, it is so much the better. However, if that is the motivation for using a new and not-yet-approved drug, it is snake oil at its worst. If the drug shows promise and ought to be explored to generate future new tools for curing cancer, it is important to explore the new drug. But the moment we say we will investigate a new drug because we have no new drug available, we are neither convinced of the ethics not clear about the science. No ethical stance can defend that attitude, for it is based on a great deal of self-delusion.

To restore the faith in medicine, there should be a clarity and dedication toward teaching. Teaching is an assertion that what we are doing is worth preserving for future generations. Teaching is, in a sense, the visible expression of faith in the system. To teach means to have clarity of thought, to understand principles, and to be open to questioning. To teach does not mean to pontificate; it does not mean to select one level of knowledge-transmission only. Our therapeutic community should continually teach itself and all outsiders who want to learn. We should teach outsiders whatever they want to learn and we should teach our own specialty students our special subset of knowledge.

To teach means to learn and to learn means to understand better. Whenever we keep a patient in the dark, we convey the message that we are too insecure to inform. To unilaterally attempt to protect patients from unpleasant knowledge is to display one's own anxieties and insecurities. To impose and order compliance is the height of internal insecurity. Our cancer centers should not be shrines shrouded in mystery, but institutions that zealously preach their knowledge so that they may not be necessary in the near future. The goal should be the cured, not the cure. If there is one place where our lack of faith is showing, it is in this area. This is also the area where we can begin to change our attitude, necessary before we are ready to admit our individual shortcomings.

The problem – the crisis in scientific medicine – is most acute in oncology, because oncology promises more to itself as well as to the world. We *can* have renewal – scientific medicine has accomplished too much to be discarded – but we must have faith in each other and ourselves before patients will believe us.

The thesis of this book is that the stresses of being a physician with traditional values of medical practice (however vaguely they are realized) can be handled as a professing Christian. This is not an attempt at reviving the priesthood of the physician. It is an attempt at stating, "healer, be healed thyself." The first level is becoming able to have faith at all, faith in what one is doing. Then faith beyond oneself, molding one's professional actions, becomes more accessible. Whatever theological perceptions shine through, come from a mixture of a Dutch Reformed – Calvinistic background, happy participation in the United Methodist Church, and wide, eclectic reading. No doubt, much fault can be found in my theology; in fact, some theologians may already have convincingly argued against my point of view. My knowledge of the Bible is not encyclopedic, and therefore I may have happily overlooked contradictions. But the central message of Christianity, the message that can be deduced from the Bible, from Church tradition, and from accepted dogma, is a salvation and grace that I believe cannot be acquired any other way.

The consequence of that belief is to feel one with other humans. In a book on the Bible, commissioned by the General Synod of the Dutch Reformed Church, this was expressed very well:

> The urgent appeal of the Gospels – which may also be a judgment – can only be made to come alive and can only become effective if [one] is prepared not just to stand over against modern man, but beside him.[10]

The Least Among Thee

Physicians must share all of their humanity and personhood with their patients, and thereby undertake to shoulder all anxieties and burdens that their patients need to unload, so that they are able to stagger along.

CHAPTER II

The Calling

The Calling

Medicine is a profession, not a science in itself. To have acquired the knowledge that allows one to practice that profession defines one as a physician in the social and legal sense. However, among all professions, physicians ought to be the last ones remaining who respond to the undiluted call for help from suffering fellow humans. There is a long-standing historical tradition for medicine to be the helping profession. I must acknowledge that the nursing profession is the same in this regard: the concepts of the nursing profession merge with those of physicians as representing helping professions.

Sir William Osler is the quintessential physician model for many doctors. He became famous in the early part of the twentieth century when medicine was in ferment in the United States and medical education as we now know it was formed. Osler thought deeply about medicine as a humanistic endeavor. He was the eighth and youngest son of a Canadian Anglican minister. Thus he was steeped in a form of thinking that was not just concrete and factual. He considered entering the ministry himself. Osler called medicine a calling. When he addressed a group of medical students, he said:

> Get your relationship clearly defined – You are in this profession as a calling, not as a business; as a calling, which exacts from you at every turn self-sacrifice, devotion, love and tenderness for your fellowmen. Once you get down to a purely business level, your influence is gone and the true light of your life is dimmed. You must work in the missionary spirit, with a breath of charity that raises you far above the petty jealousies of life.[1]

21

The Least Among Thee

Osler's personal philosophy, as can be extracted from his numerous writings, was that of a humanist rather than a scientist. He saw the practice of medicine as an art that is based on science. It is this blending of science and humanism in the practice of medicine that keeps Osler a relevant role model even today. However, he contrasted the calling of medicine with the business of medicine. While I sincerely hope that admonition will be heeded, especially in today's environment, it is not the contrast for which I am searching. More germane to my story is the contrast between a purely scientific approach, which makes the patient an object of therapy, and seeing the patient as a person in need.

The Princeton theologian, Paul Ramsey, stressed that approach to patient care in his seminal book, *The Patient as Person*.[2] Ramsey approached the physician-patient relationship as a covenant. He applied the interpretive principle of *fidelity to covenant*, with the meaning it gives to *righteousness* between human and human. There should be *faithfulness* of one human being to another. However, such concepts are often at odds with the demands, if not imperatives, of modern scientific medicine.

Modern scientific medicine generates genuine dilemmas for the physician and patient alike. Whether the patient consults the physician for a trivial but unwanted discomfort or a genuine fear of disintegration, the physician is asked to relieve the patient's perception of suffering, even when to do so, the method used is a reasoned attack on a biologically understood derangement of *physiology*. Many physicians, during their professional schooling and apprenticeships, were not trained to remain sensitive to that calling to heal the sick. Fortunately, few physicians have totally lost their sensitivity to that calling. Being a physician means responding to a call for help and thereby confronting in ourselves the willingness to help, no matter what the cost.

While medicine is a rich tradition, there is little philosophical analysis by physicians themselves. Attempts have been made – Levenson has summarized the basis for a philosophy of medicine [3] – but until recently no systematic treatise has been written on the subject. Pellegrino and Thomasma have attempted to give us one, suggesting that:

> Medicine *as* medicine is a process aimed at an *action* taken in the interest of a specific patient. Its chief aim is not discovery of the laws of nature. The end of medicine, its justifying principle, is, in the final analysis, a moral one: the "good" of a person seeking help.[4]

As Hauerwas deduced,[5] Pellegrino and Thomasma viewed medicine as a virtue. Since health is good, then medicine must be a virtue because virtue,

> … must make the right choice about the ends and purposes for which the decisions and actions are produced. Medicine must not only perform well, but also act well. It must choose what should be done to heal a particular whose good is the true and whole end of the activity.[6]

Pellegrino and Thomasma published a later book explicitly discussing medicine as a virtue.[7] But philosophical analysis of medicine as a virtue forces the argument into the abstract. True, medicine as a profession needs careful philosophical analysis. However, to be a physician is to respond to a specific need, and the general generates descriptions that ring hollow in the specific.

The temptation to discuss the virtues of medicine, or even the virtue that is medicine in the general, is a common one. The tradition of the profession called medicine evolved gradually from the priest to the practitioner of modern scientific medicine. The evolution presents a fascinating change from reliance on divine intervention to application of knowledge. However, the phenomenon "medicine" so viewed is the statistical consequence of individual behavior. But there is always a physician-patient interaction. There is always a set of common denominators applied to both patients and physicians. Patients have perceptions about health and disease that are in harmony with contemporary theological insights, scientific knowledge, and social conditions. That is true not because patients have such a vast knowledge base, but because those areas of human thought follow *per force* the tenor of the times. Physicians ply their trade within the boundaries of their knowledge and philosophy. In that sense the whole of medicine becomes a mode of dealing with the individual patient-doctor interaction. Nevertheless, this concept still avoids the antinomy of the care versus the cure. There is a tension between the community decision and the individual, between the rule and the case.

In the final analysis, medicine is an encounter between individuals – between the patient who perceives an ill and the physician who promises a healing. It is an encounter between the helper and the helped.

It would be an injustice here if I did not acknowledge that Pellegrino and Thomasma do stipulate that individual relationship.

> … The moral nature stems from the fact that patient and physician mutually enter into a healing relationship.[8]

However, they almost immediately spoil the effect by adding this:

> The healing relationship is the source of the division of labor from which physicians and patients derive rights, duties, privileges, and other forms of approval by society.[8]

Pellegrino and Thomasma also quote Babbie,[9] to show the social nature of that interaction. Accordingly, they define the interaction of individual patients and their specific physicians as the reflection of social behavior and norms. I would like to stress the converse, that medicine is the conglomerate of individual physicians' attitudes and actions.

A response to a call for help goes beyond a profession. Humans cry out for help whenever they are in enough mental agony to need support. Healing was classically embodied in the priest and the physician. Of those, priests are less the believers that they used to be. Physicians represent, in a sense, the last true helping profession.

The patient-doctor encounter is frequently, if not usually, played out against the perception of bodily illness and hoped-for cure. But there is far more behind the interaction than just biological repair. While patients ask for cure, they want restoration of health. Cure and restoration of health are not synonymous. In fact, disease and health are compatible. Curing and healing are not the same. Patients ask physicians to heal, not just to cure. Even when the disease is clearly physical, there is more to cure than removing the disease.

When I started out as a pediatric oncologist I was confronted with a concept of cancer cure that was purely biological.[10] Whenever there was no further evidence for the disease, we were tempted to call the child "cured." We could indeed boast a high percentage of prolonged survival in continuous complete unmaintained remission. But had we, in fact, created a "cured" child? In one sense, of course we had. But we did not have a "truly cured child," a child who is mentally healthy, who could function at an age-appropriate level in society. For children to be cured they have to view the world with anticipation and with an eagerness to learn what their peers are learning.[11]

Even when we do not include a metaphysical concept of disease, there is so much more to cure than eradicating disease. Cure is not just biological. How patients feel about themselves determines the cure more than does the physical reality. That does not mean that one can wish oneself well, but it does mean one can be cured even when one has had an amputation. Nor does to be cured mean that the disease is never remembered; it means that the reality of the disease is incorporated into the child's life. Once the child has had cancer, it will never disappear. That fact must not be interpreted *physically* – that is the self-defeating myth – but psychologically, because past experiences mold us into who we are.

The reality of having had cancer must be incorporated into the reality of being. This must begin early in children. We cannot wait until the experience is biologically over. Children never stop the potential for developing, and a child with cancer is still a child. We must generate an attitude towards the reality of cancer that allows the child to grow and develop normally, on par with peers, with the cancer and not in spite of the cancer,

The difference between the cured child and the truly cued child is the difference between curing and healing. Our tools as physicians are the tools for biological cure, but in curing biologically, we must also heal. It is not only children who must incorporate the reality of having had cancer into their total being; adults have the same challenge. Once one has been sick, one will never be the same again. To be healed, one must allow that new reality to be the basis for being.

Once a woman has been pregnant and has been delivered, she will always be a mother. She is not cured of pregnancy, but she has been delivered of the baby. The doctor or midwife does not cure, but assists in the delivery. The doctor is successful only if there is subsequent bonding, when the experience is positive enough for the mother to accept the child. It is true that such bonding occurs far more often than not, which might suggest that outsiders, such as the doctor, need not meddle.

Yet an analogy can be cited. We often use the equivalent of wound healing as analogy to recovery from mental anguish. However, wounds heal only when the patient is well nourished.[12] Patients recover only when they are given the environment and the encouragement necessary for healing. To use the example of the truly cured child again: "A child can learn from the environment only by choosing from what is available. If the environment allows no healthy choice, development will be warped, no matter what the child's potential."[13]

However, even a biological *and* a psychological cure are not enough. There must also be a social cure. The child, even when cured of cancer and at ease with what befell him or her, must still be reintegrated into the community. The child must be accepted as a full and equal participant in the commerce of the community, even when the child has had experiences that are so different from other children and even when the child has physical scars from the experience.[14,15]

Everyone lives in communities, variously grouped with political boundaries, limited by shared ethics, common tasks, blood ties, or friendships. Children often have little choice in the community in which they grow up. That can make reintegrating them after being declared biologically cured all the more difficult.

Physicians must extend their care beyond the science of medicine, and even beyond the care of the person. The child and the community must learn that the experience of life-threatening disease does not alter the right to full membership in the community. Physicians must remain self-effacing. They must minimize their role in the triple cure. Health should be restored without fanfare or usurping credit.

The concept "health" is, of course, an illusive one. Definitions usually address the concept "health" in the general, just as Pellegrino and Thomasma addressed the concept "medicine." Attempts have been made to define health in the context of complete mental, physical, and social well-being. That is actually a truism. Whenever one uses health, juxtaposed with social well-being the issue becomes a political one, a concern of the World Health Organization.[16] However, private health and public health are not even truly related. What makes societies healthy and what makes humans whole are not synonymous. Public health is a goal of preventive medicine. In that sense public health and private health are similar, only in one the patient is society and in the other an individual. Private health seeks to avoid the consequences of illness. But the idea of health, while usually conceptualized as absence of disease, is much more than that. Illness and health do not constitute an antinomy. One can be cured of disease and not be healthy. Conversely, one can be healthy and yet have a disease.[17] Chronic disease must be compatible with health unless we accept a notion that non-health is the norm beyond a certain age.[18]

The Least Among Thee

Because health and disease are not incompatible, they are not mutually exclusive. Few diseases are without sequelae. Even the most trivial of childhood exanthems can have a lasting effect, resulting from the behavior and reaction of the parent. Different concerns by parents about simultaneous childhood diseases in siblings can scar children for life. The effect of a disease on the state of health is therefore sometimes unpredictable. Health is an optimal state of being, socially, psychologically, and physiologically, at that age at that moment. Health is an existential concept.

Chronic disease is likewise a state of being. A chronic disease may be incurable. The gradual fading of the cardiac contractility of youth may require chronic digitalization of the elderly. That constitutes health maintenance, not disease eradication. If, for the sake of argument, we imagined cardiac transplants to be safe and available, an intervention of that conceptual magnitude would hardly constitute a restoration of health, even when it might "cure" the disease. Alternatively, if, for the sake of argument, we imagined that through a program of supervised exercise the cardiac deterioration could be postponed and compressed, that intervention would not alter the state of being of any given person at any given moment.[19] Its only effect would be to change long-range planning for the digitalis supply. The *a priori* concern with postponing a potential disease in a whole population may actually introduce non-health in non-ill persons by transferring them from the ranks of the truly healthy to the ranks of the worried well.[20]

So far, the argument is a well-known one. A person behind the illness has an idea about the illness that goes far beyond the mere physiological or pathological phenomenon. For a while there was actually a groundswell among recent medical graduates in the United States, extolling the notion, "caring' not curing." An incoming freshman to Georgetown Medical School asked the question succinctly: "Medical students: future physicians or organic mechanisms?"[21] There was some fear behind that question: not only the public opinion about medicine that he quoted,[22] but also the view medicine had of itself, one of distinct benevolence and personal business-like behavior. Joseph Garland, the long time editor of the *New England*

The Calling

Journal of Medicine, edited a book, *The Physician and his Practice.* In the foreword he wrote:

> A proper emphasis is placed on the character and personality of the physician and the standards that are expected of him – and of his wife – in relation to the two important circles in which they move: the intimate family circle and the larger community one. The fields that medicine encompasses are here defined, with discussions of the various types of activities that they offer, the necessity of hospital affiliations, the place of organization and organizations in the profession, and the physician's need for continued study – for gaining knowledge and for imparting it. Like Chaucer's clerk, gladly should he learn and gladly teach. [23]

Clearly the reemphasis on caring was sorely needed. But even in that reemphasis there was a consideration of the total society, a consideration of the many. Tisdale correctly summarized the situation when he observed:

> Physicians and philosophers have examined the practical and symbolic meanings of personal care in medicine for centuries. One conclusion reached by most scholars is that the definition and value assigned to care for the individual relate closely to the ethical ambience prevalent within the parent society. [24]

Furthermore, the caring and curing were perceived often as opposites. Some voices cried out that this seemingly excellent conceptual return to virtuous values had problems, but there were few such voices.

None of the caring-not-curing phenomenon decried modern scientific medicine. Engel observed that there was, therefore, a paradox in medicine:

> A curious paradox exists in medicine today. On the one hand we are told that never before has medicine shown more promise of being lifted beyond empiricism. Biomedical research has enormously advanced our understanding of the biochemical and genetic bases of disease, yielding a diagnostic and therapeutic armamentarium undreamed of even fifty years ago. Our medical institutions proudly boast of their excellence. Yet at the

same time medicine is charged with failure to provide adequate care, and doctors are accused of being insensitive to the needs of their patients. The medical establishment is seen as interested primarily in the perpetuation of its own power and doctors are regarded as excessively preoccupied with science, money, or both. [25]

Engel correctly observes that the problem is too much caring and not enough curing. There is science in caring also, and caring is a science for which there is too little objective knowledge as yet. Science itself is a major need in the proper development of medical care.

Black reflected on the need to be a knowledgeable physician first. He asked whether physicians must treat the whole human to provide proper medical care. He observed:

> … medicine's goal as a profession is not to prescribe the good life or even the healthy life for man. Rather, it is to free him from certain ailments, which it has characterized and tried to treat by its peculiar methods. Its goal is not describing the human ideal but rather allowing maximum freedom for each man to find his own ideal.[27]

That is overpoweringly true. The concept "health" is not the target of our knowledge; the target is the concept "biological *cure*." But we do touch human beings who ask for help. Tisdale likens physicians in one of their roles to the Good Samaritan: "The personal physician provides perceptive human support or 'Samaritanism.' This … professional function includes action termed clinical caring." [27]

However, that interpretation could be a profound misunderstanding of the idea behind Samaritanism. In an entirely different context, Gutierrez observed that the Samaritan became a helper by virtue of the one who needed him. In this interaction of helper and helped, the two merge. One takes on the burden of the helped if one extends help. As Gutierrez relates:

The Calling

The parable of the Good Samaritan ends with the famous inversion which Christ makes of the original question. They ask him, "Who is my neighbor?" And when everything seemed to point to the wounded man in the ditch on the side of the road, Christ asked, "Which of these three do you think was neighbor to the man who fell into the hands of the robbers?" (Luke 10:29, 36) The neighbor was the Samaritan who *approached* the wounded man and *made him his neighbor*. The neighbor is not he whom I find in my path, but rather, he in whose path I place myself, he whom I approach and actively seek. [28]

We are all neighbors to our patients, because they make us so. We have a skill that makes us effective. Because of our skill, we can respond effectively, but our response is called for because we are neighbors.

We need to realize our totality of being instead of just living our professional identity.[29] Just as we call the boy with hemophilia a hemophiliac, so we call the person who has knowledge and skill of nursing, a nurse. Others we call doctors, again others mental health workers, dieticians, teachers, chaplains. It is just as much a *pars pro toto* labeling to call a thinking, feeling, suffering and rejoicing human being a doctor as it is to call a boy a hemophiliac.[30]

We do that all the time, without thinking. But it creates problems in two directions: for the person who uses that term, and for the one so called, who accepts it. Those who use the term know there is a person behind the nurse, or the doctor, or the mental health worker. Therefore, the concept "doctor" becomes burdened by that image of a personhood that is preconceived by the labeler as being part of a doctor. The doctor is allowed a personality, but it is a stereotyped doctor's personality. On the other side of the problem, the label "doctor" can also be used by doctors themselves as a personality-limiting concept. Nurses, chaplains, and all of us who are professionals can do the same thing. We can hide behind being a nurse; we can hide behind being a doctor. We can become unavailable as persons, because we like the safety of our professional mask. Yet, care through availability as a person is the best care we can offer.[31]

The Least Among Thee

This could be said of any profession, any job in a cooperative effort wherein human beings interact, doing joint but assigned and defined tasks. But in the medical field the problem is compounded. Medicine touches our basic being. Taking care of the sick is a privilege; it is a task that does not produce a product but delivers a sacred service. The charge is not an object, but a totally dependent human being. Therefore, to imagine our roles in that process we must see them as part of the interactions humans have with each other whenever discomfort, suffering, anxiety, angst, loneliness, and pain are present. Medicine is a microcosm of human interactions at its most profound.

The perceptions of who we are and the basic roles we envision for ourselves and each other as human are all-prevailing and overpowering. When we are engaged in our professional role, the model and the concept of the profession fuse with the mode4ls and concepts of the whole human experience. We use imagery that is most sacred to us when suffering is the greatest. There is no doubt that we fuse nursing with motherhood and doctoring with fatherhood, with the patient as the child. The gender of the professionals is not germane to our concepts.

What defines a doctor is skill and demonstrated knowledge. Who doctors are, how they interact as human beings with the sick and how they can be friends to the patients, depend on the persons they are. Being a sensitive person does not make the doctor different in knowledge, and not necessarily more desirable as a skilled laborer in the field of medicine. Furthermore, there are so few true saints that the ideal person as doctor or as nurse is so rare as to be practically non-existent. That is just as well, because a saint is a very uncomfortable person to be around.

To be a person is the challenge. There is no difference in potential for personhood between doctors or nurses or mental health workers. To be so much of a person that we can care for others places us into "maturity" in Erikson's successive life stages.[32] We know very little about adulthood compared to what we know about childhood. We are quick to judge the appropriateness of a child's developmental maturity, but we are not very self-critical of our own adulthood. In a preface to the book *Adulthood*, Graubard observed: "Adults in contemporary society are still generally viewed in too undifferentiated a manner; all too little thought is given to the ways in which they differ from one another or from children." [33] If medical care is a microcosm of the human scene, then our vague views of adulthood further compound the problem that stem from that conceptual confusion.

However, it creates confusion only if we persist in limiting the concept "nurse" or "doctor." Of course a sick person needs to be protected, cared for, comforted, nurtured, and nourished. If the person is so sick that loved ones cannot do these things on their own anymore, we have defined a need for doctors, nurses, mental health workers, teachers, and dieticians. There is nothing wrong with that image. That is supplying the skills the patients or their families do not have.

But to be able to supply that knowledge of doctor, nurse, mental health worker, teacher, and dietician, one needs to be an adult. One needs to be secure in oneself; one needs to be able to grant personhood to the patient, whether child or adult.[34] We are all equals in the eyes of our charges because we are all caring adults who are the security of the sick. All are, to one degree or another, helpless and at our mercy. The question is, for the caregiver, indeed "Who am I?", but the answer is not, "The complete doctor." Rather, the answer is, "This person, this adult." The price we paid for the privilege of being accepted as a caring adult was learning a relevant medical skill, from dietician to doctor. There is an organization for coordinated care but no hierarchy of friendship.

It is now clear where we, as physicians, are called; because of our skills, humans call us to be their neighbors. They perceive that they need our skills, even when what they really need is to be healed. They need us to care for the whole person, not in the paternalistic sense but in the sense of shouldering their burdens.

The Least Among Thee

The doctor is indeed more than one who cures the illness or even cares for the diseased. Consider our concerns about the normalcy of the unborn child.[35] When would the newborn be so exceptional that wrongful life might ensue if the child were brought to term? How and when do we feel that the child yet to be is, in fact, normal?

To receive a new human being into the family of men is a moment of joy and a time of judgment for the parents. How that new human being was conceived and why it came into the world become the objects of scrutiny by all who will assume the joint responsibility for this new life. The care of that infant is delegated by society to the parents, but it is ultimately for the common good, for independent participation, that the child will be raised.

To conceive, carry, and birth a new life creates a time of anxiety and hope. Without anxiety the child would be brought into the world thoughtlessly, and without hope the child would not bring the joy the parents deserve,

Unfortunately, in many parents there is little hope. Anxiety so often out-weighs hope. The complementarity of anxiety and hope as part of the same mature perception is rarely consciously, or even subconsciously, understood by the parents.[36] The anxiety is learned before the hope is realized. This anxiety is conceptualized into concern about whether the child can cope in the family of men, whether the child can have the happiness without which the parents conceive existence to be intolerable misery. But the concept is verbalized and concretized by asking, "Will my child be normal?" The concept normalcy in that context embraces coping, thinking, the soul – but the question is asked in the concrete and is considered as form, function, body. There is still a lot of *mens sana in corpore sano* in or collective thinking.

But who, then, is normal? Ultimately there is only one normal that we can rely on: we ourselves are normal. But that is not an adequate or secure touchstone. We rarely understand who we are, and therefore we cannot translate our own mental health and physical satisfaction, if indeed we have such normalcy, into a generalization for all. Actually, we frequently have doubts about our own normalcy and worry about our mental state. When we have such doubts and concerns, we translate our doubts about our normalcy into concerns over our physical well-being. We go to the doctor with questions about our physical health when, unvoiced and unrealized, our concern is about our normalcy of being.

It is no wonder, then, that we translate our anxiety about normalcy of being for the newly conceived lives into judgments about their physical normalcy. Most people think that determination of physical normalcy solves the problem, and that objective decisions can be made through medical judgments. However, even in medicine the concept of normalcy is very difficult to concretize. A patient who goes to the doctor with complaints is considered sick until illness is ruled out by exclusion. The routine physical examination attempts to find disease of which the patient is not aware. However, to declare a patient healthy, normal, the physician is likely to say, "I cannot find anything wrong and the tests all came back 'normal'." Just as we objectify and concretize normalcy of spirit by looking for assurance of normalcy of body (the physical examination), we try to establish normalcy of the body by looking for normalcy of physiology and chemistry (the tests). By that time we are two steps removed from the primary concern.

When the concern about being well, normal, healthy, is that of the patients about themselves, the distinction between health and disease is even more imperfectly perceived. No matter what seemed to be the question, the calling of a physician is not to be the curer of the disease. That is the skill of the physician. By acquiring that skill the physician has made it imperative to respond to the call of the patients that will come. The physician has made a commitment to as yet unspoken calls. The physician has become the neighbor of the patient because the patient stepped in his path. By being the neighbor, the physician can heal.

To be a neighbor one has to see a person. As Kierkegaard said:

The Least Among Thee

He who feeds the poor but yet is not victorious over his own mind in such a way that he calls this feeding a feast sees in the poor and unimportant only the poor and unimportant. He who gives a feast sees in the poor and unimportant his neighbors.[37]

The doctors, who see in the patient only a sick person, are not loving their neighbor. To love their neighbor they need to see a person in need, a human being for whom they offer all they have to offer in their own humanity, the feast of shared suffering.

Healing is a biblical concept. Remember the story of the ten lepers:

> And it came to pass, as he went to Jerusalem, that he passed through the midst of Samaria and Galilee. As he entered into a certain village, there met him ten men who were lepers, which stood afar off: and they lifted up their voices, and said, 'Jesus, Master, have mercy on us.' And when he saw them he said unto them, 'Go show your selves unto the priests.' And it came to pass, that, as they went, they were cleansed. And one of them, when he saw that he was healed, turned back and with a loud voice glorified God, and fell down on his face at his feet, giving thanks: and he was a Samaritan. And Jesus, answering, said, 'Were there not ten cleansed? But where are the nine? There are not found that returned to give glory to God, save this stranger.' And he said to him, 'Arise, go thy way: thy faith has made thee whole.'" [38]

As physicians we do more for patients than curing their disease. It is that conviction and that realization that heals.

To be sick is normal.[39] It is the reaction to illness that requires healing, while curing the illness as best we can and the patient's body lets us. The act of healing is a remarkable phenomenon. Remember the old biblical story:

> And now some men brought him a paralyzed man lying on a bed. Seeing their faith, Jesus said to the man, "Take heart my son, your sins are forgiven." At this some of the lawyers said to themselves, "This is blasphemous talk." Jesus knew what they were thinking, and said, "Why do you harbor these

evil thoughts? Is it easier to say, 'Your sins are forgiven,' or to say, 'Stand up and walk'? But to convince you that the Son of Man has the right to forgive sins – he turned to the paralyzed man – "Stand up, take your bed and go home." Thereupon the man got up, and went off home. The people were filled with awe at the sight, and praised God for granting such authority to men.[40]

The calling to be a physician is the calling to be a person who can respond to a very special call for help. The calling is to heal, but in order to convince the patient that physicians have to right to heal, they must first attempt to cure.

This calling is very different from the undertaking to consider the total patient scientifically. To answer the call, however, the physician need not be doctor, priest, social worker, nurse, dietician, and philosopher all at once. Answering the call means recognizing that one's patient is your neighbor and, in the special encounter that illness brings, a very wounded neighbor. Physicians are not called to restore health, but to heal. David Rogers used the phrase, "The doctor himself must become the treatment. He said:

> An illness ... is a *human* event. It is a grouping of discomforts, dysfunctions, anxieties, changes in feeling state and in the ability to function, which occur in a *person*. Illness is, in essence, an interaction of a particular person with a particular disease. It is an event in the course of a human life. It is often of great importance and often profoundly influenced by the background, life style, and temperament of the individual who is experiencing it. It is embedded in the trappings of concerns, responsibilities, hopes, and fears of that special and unique and particular person. Thus an illness is ultimately to be understood not in scientific but in human terms.[41]

To be a physician who heals one has to be a person who can share that profound human experience. Curing the disease changes the human experience, and curing alone would leave a void unless healing of the wounds inflicted by the disease occurs, or unless healing of the wounds, imagined to be a disease, is accomplished.

The Least Among Thee

In order to be a neighbor to all those who are afflicted, one must love one's neighbor. Kierkegaard summarized this calling:

> One's neighbor is one's equal. One's neighbor is not the beloved for whom you have passionate preference, nor your friend for whom you have passionate preference. Nor is your neighbor, if you are well educated, the well educated person with whom you have cultural equality – for with your neighbor you have before God the equality of humanity. Nor is your neighbor one who is of higher social status than you, that is, insofar as he is of higher social status he is not your neighbor, for to love him because of his higher status than you can easily be preference and to that extent self-love. Nor is your neighbor one that is inferior to you, that is, insofar as he is inferior he is not your neighbor, for to love one because he is inferior to you can easily be partiality's condescension and to that extent self-love. No, to love one's neighbors means equality. It is encouraging in your relationship to people of distinction that in them you *shall* love your neighbor. In relation to those inferior it is humbling that in them you are not to love the inferior but *shall* love your neighbor. If you do this there is salvation, for you *shall* do it. Your5 neighbor is every man, for on the basis of distinction he is not your neighbor, nor on the basis likeness to you as being different from other men. He is your neighbor on the basis of equality with you before God, but this equality absolutely every man has, and he has it absolutely.[42]

Given that equality, to be a physician is to share the burden of the illness with the patient. The calling of a physician is to be the sensitive Samaritan to the wounded fellow traveler who makes that physician his neighbor. To have the skills of a physician is to be able to respond, as a neighbor, to that very special call for help.

The calling to be a physician is a calling to help the ones most needy, but not because the physician thereby acquires power and authority. For, to act on that power and out of that authority, is to that extent, self-love. To be a physician is to act from the knowledge that every patient has equality to the physician and has it absolutely, because we are of the same flesh and spirit before God.

CHAPTER III

Rebellion

Rebellion

To become a physician means to acquire a vast personal knowledge and an even vaster knowledge pool, to which medical students and house staff in training learn to gain access. Finally, to become a physician means to stress continuing education, because the physician learns that medical knowledge is a process, ever-increasing and improving.

That is true not just for academic physicians, but for all physicians. It is instructive to quote from the catalogue of the University of Texas Medical School at Houston:

> The primary and overriding objective of the University of Texas Medical School at Houston is the education of physicians for practice. In addition to the prevention and cure of disease and the alleviation of physical and emotional suffering, the modern physician remains as responsible as ever as advisor and counselor to his [sic] in matters pertaining to maintaining physical and mental health.

> To achieve this goal, the School selects a broadly representative group of well-prepared, highly motivated, intellectually able, and emotionally stable young people from a variety of experiential, cultural, social and economic backgrounds and offers them personalized educational experiences which will encourage them to understand the biological and scientific bases of modern medicine; to understand the cultural and social forces which shape modern medicine, and the role of physicians in that culture; to gain cognitive, manual, and interpersonal skills necessary for the physician; and to gain skill in problem solving. This process is seen as encompassing more than the student's four years in medical

school. It is assumed all graduates will seek further supervised medical training. It is further assumed that for the entire duration of his career each physician will expend continuing effort in maintaining his skills. The primary objective of the School includes educational experiences in graduate and continuing medical education.[1]

The intertwining of knowledge, skill and humane medicine are a continuing theme as the medical curriculum is presented:

> To achieve this primary objective four additional objectives are necessary: A University Medical School; Provision of Health Services; Community Involvement; Health Care Delivery.[2]

In its descriptions the University Medical School recognizes knowledge and science as continuing needs for the physician of the future:

> The creation of cultural, medical, educational and scientific resources of the first rank with the characteristics and attitudes of the university is the first of these objectives. Society rightfully expects of its universities a concern for the future, explicit examination of the issues of today, aggressive search for new knowledge and, in the case of the medically oriented schools of the university, a focus on human health, disability and disease. The school has an unquestionable commitment to science: biomedical, physical, and social. Every effort has been made to select strong scientific leadership in important biomedical fields where the challenges are both large and susceptible to answer. For over a century laboratory research has been medicine's most effective and powerful agent for change. There is no evidence that this will not continue to be true, and the School attests to this conviction in its faculty and educational programs.[3]

All medical schools, to varying degrees, repeat these promises. The emphasis on primary or tertiary care may vary. The perceived function of the school may be skewed to one or the other possible model of the physician. However, all acknowledge medical science as a necessary and powerful tool in the physician's armamentarium.

Rebellion

The moral and ethical dilemmas that are posed by science's ever increasing knowledge and capabilities are continually confronting us. Life-support systems are postponing the moment of death; definitions of death are being rewritten, and undoubtedly will change again in the future. Little of this needs documentation; bookstores and libraries abound with information and documented debate on the subject. Such information and technology vastly increase the power with which the physician can combat disease. It does no good to decry them.

We must, however, retain a healthy awareness of the human being's uncontrollable propensity to corruption. A tool is only the extension of the user. A respirator is a tool that allows mechanical ventilation in place of manual ventilation. Although the respirator is a great refinement, the choice of whether to use or discontinue it raises a dilemma for the user. The good or evil embodied in the respirator is only the good or evil of the one who controls it. The respirator represents no new creation, no new insight into life and death. The respirator is morally, ethically, and theologically neutral. The ability to perform an abortion safely, or the opposite, to keep a conceptus alive *ex utero* at ever earlier times, also falls into the category of technological achievements that are in themselves neutral.[4]

There is power in medicine. We have the capabilities of curing diseases that were until recently the dreaded scourges of humankind. There was a time when Pellagra severely afflicted populations. Physicians recognized its four "*D*"s: dermatitis, diarrhea, dementia, and death. At one time the approach to the disease was psychiatric, where the overwhelming influence of Freudian theory made it impossible to assume that such patients with pellagra were not psychogenically psychotic.[5] The discovery of nicotinic acid as a vitamin and of the biochemical relationship of tryptophan and nicotinic acid changed all that. Pellagra is not yet totally understood, but today it can be cured when it occurs and prevented when it threatens.[6] It is true power to prevent a preventable death and to treat the human misery that pellagra presented.

Many of the endemic scourges of mankind have been so conquered. Plague is no longer the decimator of populations that it once was. The disease still occurs sporadically in New Mexico, but the danger that a patient faces in the United States is more that physicians may not recognize it rather than that the disease is inherently dangerous.[7] Tuberculosis is now a preventable and curable disease. It was only a short time ago that it was clothed in myths to the same degree that AIDS is now.[8] It is true that our attempts at treatment have given rise to treatment-resistant tuberculosis. Similar challenges are arising in other infectious diseases as well. However, that does not change the basic argument that physicians exercise power over disease and sometimes are clearly successful.

Fries, a physician, actually suggested that, with advanced age, persons will be free of disease and die a natural death: a sudden interruption of functions from old age.[9] That view clearly illustrates the presupposition that disease is definable, and, of course, in many instances biological disease is indeed definable. When disease is the consequence of an external agent, such as microbes, viruses, or trauma, the disease is ultimately defined by its cause. The extrapolation that therefore all disease is definable is not an unreasonable concept for the future. Even before that presumed ideal is reached, there is no doubt that physicians will acquire more skills, more tools, and more drugs to combat the effect of illness on the body. Fries found that concept a pleasant one.

The American Psychological Association saw a more frightening specter. Peele stated in the abstract of a paper, entitled "Reductionism in the Psychology of the Eighties":

> A growing consensus is emerging that the best hope for understanding and dealing with psychological problems lies with work being done in genetics, biology, and the neurosciences. Research in the neurosciences, especially, is expected to revolutionize the treatment of mental disorders in the coming years. The public is kept abreast of progress in this field in article after article in mass publication periodicals. Moreover, psychologists appear so eager to accept neurological and biochemical explanations for behavior that psychology is in danger of losing its status as an independent body of knowledge. This reductionist trend of thought, as well as having major

scientific implications, affects popular attitudes toward self regulation in key areas of human functioning. Yet, not only has biological and neurological research *not* explained basic aspects of human behavior and mental disorder, it has fundamental problems in attempting such explanations.[10]

Peele then proceeds to present what he perceives to be a "psychology that accepts and accounts for subjective human experience as a counterpoise to the reductionists' thrust." Peele correctly states that "the appeal of reductionists' thinking lies in its concreteness and its conciseness." [11] We do in fact consider mental illness an illness on the medical model. That would allow a solution, a cure on the medical model as well. Thomas Szasz has for years railed against that concept, calling it "The Myth of Mental Illness." [12]

But this reductionism, so hopefully espoused by Fries and so decried by Peele and Szasz, is used by physicians primarily to shore up their authority. Most physicians do hear, or at least have heard, the calling. They may not have heard it in the extreme challenge of a Christianity that allows only full commitment, but they most certainly perceived the need for healing, because they perceive a suffering behind the disease that is far beyond the biological impact. There is no doubt that the special skill of the physician is necessary to alleviate that suffering. To apply that skill is to take up battle against the disease. Physicians ask with all fellow humans the same question, "Why all this suffering?"

Vaux describes the Western view of illness as having evolved through three stages: tradition, experiment, and renovation.[13] He calls the traditional concept "illness as punishment." The concept that "research will eventually conquer all disease" he calls the experiment. In renovation, Vaux sees a curbing of the technical skills of the experiment with the supernatural wisdom of tradition.

His analysis, however, does not help in the confrontation between neighbors: the wounded patient and the Samaritan physician. The first emotion the Samaritan may have felt was a rage against the inhuman robbers who so wounded the traveler. But who inflicts disease on the patient? We view plagues as the scourge of God, a punishment of the way humans act, inflicted upon the individual. We still feel at ease with Father Paneloux's sermon in Camus', *The Plague:*

> If today the plague is in your midst, that is because the hour has struck for taking thought. The just man need have no fear, but the evildoer has good cause to tremble. For plague is the flail of God and the world His threshing floor and implacably He will thresh out his harvest until the wheat is separated from the chaff.[14]

And yet, we cannot be physicians and accept such a view of suffering and punishment. We are called by our patients to be their neighbor. Vaux reflected on *The Plague* by Camus:

> You will recall that the doctor in *The Plague* hangs in there after all the others have pulled out as the plague decimates the community. He does not know why he does not believe anything, but he knows he must stay by these people who are hurting and dying. As I understand the Bible and in particularly the Book of Job, our humanity means nothing more or less than shaking one's fist in the face of God, demanding that He live out his righteousness. That is what Job does, that is what it is to be a human being. The way we express our resistance to death and disease – is by doing the things we have invested our whole lives in – caring, standing by, getting up the next morning, and coming in and doing it again. That is our resistance and that is our affirmation of hope.[15]

In this struggle against disease the physician has a skill, acquired in learning. The patients call for help because of the skill we have. Physicians help, and help again, but they do have anger against Him who inflicted those wounds.

To have the skill of a physician is to acquire a certain power over disease. The physician also possesses authority. The physician has actual authority by being licensed by the State to do such procedures and prescribe such drugs as are deemed necessary to remove disease. That in itself creates the burden of being a physician. There is much more to it, however. Not only do physicians have such legally constituted authority, but they also practice an authority that is perceived by patients as morally desirable. Hauerwas discusses that concept of authority, but shies away from the perception the physician has of that authority when confronted with a calling.[16] After receiving the call, the physician's first reaction is anger. The physician commands authority to rectify the injustice, making ever greater effort to conquer disease. When I asked, "What shall we do? Stand up and take on God?" Ken Vaux answered, "Yes, it is exactly what we are meant to do."[17]

Accordingly, research in medicine is pursued with ever greater passion. We are so affronted by the perception of injustice that we want to command the tools to combat the overt sin of suffering the disease. Pierre Teilhard de Chardin wrote:

> We must struggle against death with all our force, for it is our fundamental duty as living creatures.

He went on to say:

> But when by virtue of a state of things ... death takes up, we must experience the paroxysm of faith in life that causes us to abandon ourselves to death as to falling into a greater life.[18]

But when a patient clearly has not accepted that "state of things," but calls for help, because resignation has not yet dulled the suffering of disease, the physician must actively combat the illness, and passively reflect on the meaning of health and disease. The authority that the physician commands is not sufficient to exorcise all suffering. Physicians receive a mandate to do research, and physicians receive a promise in research even now.

The promise, and the pay-off, in research are easily demonstrated. So much emphasis has been placed on the dilemmas at the edges of life that new technology has generated, that we forget the near miraculous progress that medical research and consequent technology have made. After the assassination attempt on President Reagan in 1981, many comparisons were made with other assassination attempts on other presidents. Stevens compares the course of President Garfield's illness after the assassination attempt in 1881 with that of Reagan a century later:

> Throughout the course of his 80-day illness Garfield received no intravenous fluids, no hyper-alimentation, no blood transfusions, no roentgenograms, no antibiotics, and no definitive surgery. Anyone alone might well have saved his life.[19]

Stevens continued later:

> It is interesting to speculate what 1981 medicine might have done for President Garfield. It is not hard to imagine what would happen to a 70-year old president shot in the lung in 1881. Without modern American medicine, President Reagan would have swiftly followed the course of Garfield, Lincoln, and McKinley.[20]

Stevens decried the lack of improvement in American society in the century between the attacks on Garfield and Reagan, but he correctly stated:

> Medicine, at least, has improved substantially in the past century, and President Reagan and thousands of other trauma victims are alive today because of it. The next time someone criticizes modern medicine, remind them how it saved Reagan's life. And tell them what happened to Garfield.[21]

Not just presidents, but people of all walks of life, have benefited from medical research. Not just trauma victims but sufferers of all diseases are being helped. Research and technology directed at trauma medicine does not have the urgency that research against pure disease does. The anger against the assassin is understandable and manageable. But rarely is there an assassin behind the purely medical and surgical disease. The anger must be directly vaguely elsewhere, unless we indeed admit anger at God.

Rebellion

The imperative is therefore perceived: we must do research. Research is a mode to alleviate suffering, if not now in this patient then later in future patients. To expedite research we must, on occasion, do the research on patients themselves. In fact, many physicians argue that experimental therapy is the best therapy because it represents the best thought that medicine has to offer at any given time.[22] In a profound sense this is true. The eradication of disease, when that is the sole target, may well be best approached by experiment. The individual doctor who has the responsibility entrusted by that individual patient may well need to battle with research approaches. It may be the only way in which the physician can command the trust in being healed that the patient needs.[23]

This drive to take on God in battling disease through research was soon translated into a social mandate that was the result of an extreme extrapolation but which gave rise to a codified behavior not unlike the elaborate rules of chivalry. The National Commission for the Protection of Human Subjects, in its recommendations on Institutional Review Boards, started out:

> The ethical conduct of research involving human subjects requires a balance of society's interest in protecting the rights of the subjects and in developing knowledge that can benefit the subjects of society as a whole.[24]

The whole bio-ethical enterprise that was spawned by the National Commission focused largely on society's needs versus the individual's rights. Little attention was given to the physicians urge to battle disease at all costs. To be a physician and to truly be the neighbor of one's patient, to truly share the burden of the suffering, is difficult to the point of engendering rebellion.

Vaux, in his book on medical ethics, claims that we are truly taking on God, that we are usurping His powers. Vaux states:

> The fall of man is seen in its full biblical ambivalence. It is both fortunate and tragic. It lifts him to an unsurpassed height of science and prescience.

It takes him to the brink of hell. He gains mastery over unexplorable mystery. He becomes the maker and giver of life. He is summoned to "come and play God." [25]

He goes on to say:

We ask in our excitement and terror, "Shall we make and remake man? Shall we tamper with the building blocks of life? Shall we play God?" Perhaps we decided affirmatively long ago when, as Prometheus and Pandora, we just controlled fire or took a drug. We do it again and again when we treat a wound or build a dike or receive an inoculation. Today, although the question is given profound dimension, we are asking an old question, "Should man play God?" [26]

The phrase "Should doctors play God?" is the frequently unwritten but often quoted question posed to all groups debating, considering or contemplating the impact of modern knowledge upon medical practice.[27] The question is almost always asked in a tone that allows only the response, "Of course not." After that, ethical analysis proceeds in such a way that one can discern how such an arrogant stance by doctors can be avoided or averted. It must be clear that there is a concept behind that question that implies a negative connotation behind "play." Playing is envisioned as impersonating, pretending to be what one is not. It also implies that the play will have permanent consequences; that play is more than make-believe.

The concept of play is in fact enormously complex. The word is used as a noun, a transitive verb, and an intransitive verb. It is a performance, the script of a performance; it can denote a serious act or a jest, a pronouncement or a pun. The definition used in the question "Should doctors play God?" is "to act the part in real life," one of the seventy four definable uses.

North Carolina allergist Claude Frazier edited a book titled by our phrase. In that book Mrs. Billy Graham wrote a foreword:

Rebellion

> If I were an actress who was going to play, let's say, Joan of Arc, I would learn all there is to learn about Joan of Arc. And if I were a doctor or anyone else trying to play God, I would learn all I could about God. When one does this, one learns one cannot play God. One can only obey Him or disobey Him.[28]

There is another concept embodied in the verb "to play": to exercise or employ oneself in diversion – where playing is not altogether serious. This form of play is more associated with children, and is pleasurable. For children, however, these two concepts are in fact intertwined. Children play very seriously. They act out the world they do not understand. They imitate their parents to understand what it must be like to be parents. Play is "the child's natural medium of self-expression."[29] When that element of children's play is the focus of observation by an adult, we have non-directive play therapy. As Axline says:

> Since play is the natural medium for self-expression, the child is given the opportunity to play out his accumulated feelings of tension, frustration, insecurity, aggression, fear, confusion.[30]

All child's play has an element of that unburdening of pent-up emotions and struggling with understanding. Much of children's playing is a non-directive play therapy. But so is some of the play of adults. It is important to view the question, "Should doctors play God??" with that concept of play in mind. It is not inconceivable that there are times in the development of the mature physician that a period of "playing God" is necessary to reach an understanding of a God who is so infinitely more incomprehensible to an adult than is the inscrutable and capricious parent to a child.

Playing God as a doctor implies acting powerfully, authoritatively, knowingly, and presciently in the face of suffering and death. God is inscrutable when suffering touches the human. For a while Job could say:

> The Lord gives and the Lord takes away,
> Blessed be the name of the Lord.[31]

The Least Among Thee

But that did not suffice and, ultimately, Job had to say to the Lord, who proclaims His majesty:

> I know that thou canst do all things and that no purpose is beyond thee. But I have spoken of great things which I have not understood, things too wonderful for me to know. I know of thee then only by report, but now I see thee with my own eyes. Therefore I melt away; I repent in dust and ashes. [32]

Job may have understood, but most modern humans who hear Job find such a God inscrutable, capricious, arbitrary, and frightening. Emily Dickenson must have felt that power of an inscrutable God very keenly when she wrote:

> Heavenly father – take to thee
> The supreme iniquity
> Fashioned by thy candid hand
> In a moment contraband –
> Though to trust us – seem to us
> More respectful – We are dust –
> We apologize to thee
> For thine own Duplicity. [33]

Few of us have the power of words granted Emily Dickinson, and few of us would even then express ourselves that rebelliously to a capricious God who brings suffering to the seemingly undeserving. In the face of all such illness and suffering, the perception of the hand of God demands play therapy for adults as much as the little child needs play therapy to understand the perceived hurt and suffering inflicted by capricious and inscrutable parents.

Children overstep allowable bounds in their play. So do adults: in playing God, in fact, doctors can overstep their bounds. But that is not at all frequent, and rarely occurs in the context of play as here understood. There are times when doctors make a decision because a decision needs to be made. Sometimes doctors struggle with God as Jacob did and may call, "I will not let you go unless you bless me," [34] and sometimes doctors can

Rebellion

limp away from that encounter, saying "I have seen God face to face and my life is spared." [35] That kind of an encounter, a struggle of such biblical magnitude, may be called play in modern man's imagery, but it is a deadly serious encounter. Once that struggle is joined, play is over. The Roman poet Horace said it succinctly:

> Be not ashamed of playing, unless you would not stop.[36]

To play God, to try to fathom God's unplumbable capriciousness, is within the best concept of mental health for doctors. Not to do so is to be an automaton, to be a mentally handicapped adult, as surely as the child is handicapped who is never allowed to act independently or to play out the adult world.

The doctor does play God. Doctors must play God to learn – playing God is trying out our Prometheus instinct. To be adult is to know that not all potential can be actualized. Play is serious because it is not play acting. Through playing God, the doctor tries to understand God. Through playing God, doctors learn the limits of their power. Only through playing God will they learn to accept God.

What choices does the doctor have? The teenager Hamlet did not understand adult behavior. In his dilemma he did not know what to do, and he acted out all possible scenarios. Is not his question the universal one of the physician who struggles with the role of God's hand in the illness of his patient?

> Whether it is nobler in the mind to suffer
> The slings and arrows of outrageous fortune,
> Or to take arms against a sea of troubles,
> And by opposing end them? [37]

Doctors try both and decide. That is how a child chooses and that is how the adult, as a child before God, chooses it. To learn to understand is not resignation but wisdom. To grow and act like an adult is proper. But the struggle with God, the attempt at understanding God, is not wrong; it is medicine in the best tradition. To truly understand God is not possible; to think one does makes one presume to be a priest and not a doctor.

There are many humans who play God by becoming doctors. So frequently we serve our own needs. But a child who plays well, who experiments profitably with the adult world, would be a sought-after playmate, much to be desired as a friend by children and their parents alike. All persons ought to seek out those doctors who play God, who try to understand, who imagine to the best of their abilities what God did and would do, and who test the limits of their own authority. We should not interfere with such play, but join in. We have much to learn.

When children play, they do not consciously acknowledge the purpose and the role. In fact, when they do, the effect is lost to a degree. An analogy can be found in the use of fairy tales. Bruno Bettelheim discussed that subject in detail in his delightful book, *The Uses of Enchantment*. There are many deep meanings in fairy tales that help children deal with basic existential problems like sibling rivalry, separation anxiety, and early puberty. Repetitious hearing of such stories helps the child work through the problems. However, Bettelheim observes:

> Even if a parent should guess correctly why his child has become involved emotionally with a given tale, this knowledge is best kept to oneself. The young child's most potent experiences and reactions are largely subconscious and should remain so until he reaches a much more mature age and understanding.[38]

So it is with playing parent. What is played is real, why it is played is subconscious. Furthermore, the child plays parent, not mommy or daddy, and only that part of being parent is of concern. Doctors play God in the sense that they subsume responsibility for a single parent as part of their total responsibility and consider their power in the face of God. When

Rebellion

Hamlet became conscious of his struggle, his play became staged, and his anxieties became incapacitating:

> And thus the native hue of resolution
> Is sicklied o'er with the pale cast of thought.[39]

After that, one cannot anymore solve conflicts by play.

Play can get out of hand, and play can generate more, rather than less, anxiety. The disturbed child can repeat the same game over and over again. But when the concept is mastered, the problem is solved, and the play is over. Play makes the child grow. When the problem is solved the child has matured. The wisdom, the understanding, will not prevail consciously. So will it be when the doctor is playing wisely; understanding of God, or realizing it is alright not to know, will prevail, and decisions will be made humbly.

The disturbed child usually keeps play in bounds, and even the doctor keeps his playing God in bounds. The constraint is in part peer pressure, in part parental guidance (for the child) and mentor guidance (for the doctor). But more pressing is the concept behind the play. To play God, one must have an idea of God, and an idea that disturbs. The very need for playing implies a belief in God, or concern about God.

No analogy can be exhaustively stretched. There is, however, a greater element of Prometheus in us than we admit. The child wants little more than to become an adult. There is little desirable about childhood in a child's eyes. All of us want in some part to be God and to act as God. We stand in line from snake to Eve to Adam to us. To understand what that means we play at it. That is healthy. That is, to a large degree, what has made medicine what it is today.

Unfortunately, we reserve the question, "Should doctors play God?" precisely for those situations in which doctors do not play God in the childlike sense anymore, nor even in the sense of being an actor, but in the sense of taking the place of God. The actor fuses with the part, the play is over, and identity is destroyed. Faust sold his soul, Jekyll and Hyde merge. We are right to be frightened of that specter.

Often, the serious play in medicine will not be recognized by the ones who ask the question of whether doctors should be allowed to play God and the public's narcissistic[40] concerns will remain served. However, we may thereby lose a vital insight into medicine's behavior.

Once we become mature, play is over. Maturity demands realization of self. Adulthood can be reached. Adulthood is the most stressful of all human development stages. Erikson counterpoised on the adulthood stage generativity *versus* stagnation or self-absorption. Generativity includes productivity and creativity, but it is also concerned with guiding the next generation. The later stage of maturity, including old age, counterpoises ego-integrity *versus* despair.[41] Here is the real analogy to the mature adult doctor, who listens to the call for help of the patient, and does not despair about the inability to challenge the reality of the illness.

The virtue of the first age of adulthood is care, and of the maturity stage is wisdom. The ideal for the physician is care with wisdom. Erikson himself once said he was not "satisfied with wisdom because to some it seemed to mean a too strenuous achievement for each and every old person."[42] But physicians have a calling that is not just for each and every person. To a degree physicians cannot wait for wisdom to come in old age. Their rebellion must come early; their playing God must be completely successful to allow generativity and ego-integrity to occur.

Erikson himself defined wisdom as:

> ... the detached and yet active concern with life itself, in the face of death itself, which maintains and conveys the integrity of experience in spite of the disdain over human failings and the dread of ultimate non-being.[43]

Rebellion

This is not wisdom for the patient but about the self. This wisdom is no different from the general wisdom to be achieved by all humans; only the circumstances of the physician make the question both acutely poignant and readily open to misconstruing.

Erikson counterpoises two elements. The virtue "care" in adulthood must be achieved by the physician before "wisdom" can be achieved. Each of Erikson's stages must be mastered before the next one can be incorporated. At each stage there will be a fork in the road. The adult physician must proceed through generativity to achieve integrity. If not, stagnation or self-absorption will ensue. There is no escaping that the patient-doctor relationship brings a responsibility to the doctor that is a burden to carry far beyond our independent capabilities.

A practicing physician gave us another powerful metaphor, that of Abraham and Isaac:

> You bring him here
> To this aseptic altar,
> Isaac again; fear
> Tumbling fear.
>
> And I, conscripted god,
> Allowed no qualm or grief;
> No sign – no serpent rod;
> Offer up my silent prayer.[44]

A call from God is embodied in the presence of disease. There is little the patient or family can do but to answer that call. The patients are brought to the physician, who is the only one who may save the patient Isaac from sacrifice to death. Patients and their families come to the physician with "Fear and Trembling."[45] The physician must respond. It is no wonder that, after trying to understand the God who could call Abraham to bring Isaac to the altar, one emotion can be anger, a fight against the disease.

The Least Among Thee

Bartholome once pointed out the martial approach we use to diseases such as cancer. Speaking at a conference on the care of the child with cancer, he observed:

> As my research assistant and I read the material we had gathered, we were repeatedly struck by what we have called the "military imagery." Cancer is the enemy. The pediatric oncologist, and the vast spectrum of professionals who have come to research centers, have declared war on childhood cancer. New drugs, as they are developed, are added to the arsenal of weapons. The radiotherapy branch is ardently searching for better ways to focus the killing x-ray beam on the foreign cells. The cancer is perceived as a state of anarchy, and therapy is designated to eradicate this anarchical system. The abnormal tissue is often referred to as "target tissue." Cancer is to be cut out, destroyed, killed, and at all costs – physical, mental, spiritual, not to mention economic – eradicated. The agents developed to do the killing are toxins, poisons, and anti-metabolites. Obviously, in such a war, the end point is total and lasting destruction of the enemy. The child's body is the battlefield.[46]

He asked:

> As the scope of concerns enlarges beyond that of a thorough kill, those who conduct this war discover that comprehensive care of the child with cancer involves more than a "clean kill." Are those men and women who answered the call to arms against childhood cancer able to see that conceptualizing cancer as a war has made them blind to the child as a patient? Are these warriors willing, or able, to give up this abstraction to deal concretely with the lived illness of the children? With this attitude can a "therapeutic community" be established? My impression is that the battle continues to be waged, and that many of those involved have little or no time for the children. They still take a back seat to the needs and demands of research.[47]

Yet, there are physicians who genuinely feel that anger at the robbers would not have helped the traveler in the ditch. The Good Samaritan did not fight decay in law and order, but paid for the housing and care of his self-accepted charge. He did not conduct research on trauma for the good of society so that the next victim could be more expeditiously helped.

Rebellion

Undoubtedly, such research could have helped the physician greatly, and there is a great need for such knowledge. But to conduct research out of anger and frustration is to avoid heeding the totality of the call. There will come a day wherein we shall say with the psalmist:

> Who is aware of his unwritten sins?
> Cleanse me of any secret fault,
> Hold back thy servant also from sins of self will
> Lest they get the better of me.
> Then I shall be blameless
> and innocent of any transgression.
> May all that I say and think be acceptable to thee,
> O Lord, my soul and my redeemer.[48]

Physicians are indeed the executors of God's will. Physicians are their patient's neighbor. But more than that, they are seen also as their patient's redeemer. Whatever images patients use to describe their disease and its cause, all contain an element of fear of self-annihilation and a concept of God.

Once their rebellion is over and the anger dissipated, physicians undertake the role of their calling. Some of those physicians will indeed progress to adulthood. The price they pay for that maturation is very great. To be an adult with the calling of a physician is a very precarious position indeed.

CHAPTER IV

Acknowledgment and Guilt

Acknowledgment and Guilt

When, as a physician, one is faced with being the Samaritan to the patient-neighbor, one must also share his or her burdens. There is no alternative. The physician must not only be responsible for treating the illness, but must also share all the frightening meaning the patient places on the illness. Patients ask to be helped, and to try to help is to promise help. To promise help and not be able to deliver can be acceptable only if a genuine attempt at healing is made. Whatever guilt the patient carries from having been sick must be accepted by the physician for failing to relieve the patient's guilt by removing the disease. If we can't deliver a ram in place of Isaac we are guilty of Isaac's death. That guilt weighs very heavily. That guilt is integral to our mature generativity and integrity. To be a true physician is to share all the illness with the patient – not just the physical symptoms, not even just the social impact, but the whole anxiety that the disease generates, the angst that is the illness.

Often the patient sees the disease as the cause of fear, as the physical sign of punishment for past transgressions. At all times the patient sees the disease as an unwanted intruder that threatens the total being. By being asked to take away the disease, the physician cannot avoid involvement with the total being of the patient.

To be a healer is to carry the wounds of suffering. Nouwen used the term, "The Wounded Healer." He was speaking of ministers, who are also approached by persons in need who have all the same ontological anxieties. But unlike physicians, ministers lack the ability and skill to promise relief.

The Least Among Thee

The disease is the language the patient uses to explain those anxieties, and the physician accepts that basis of dialogue. But the language has deep meaning. The concepts behind the statement that one feels ill are profound. Unless the physician incorporates the same concept in the words, communication fails and the patient is not helped. To speak of the practice of medicine as the ideal, and not of the individual encounter is to avoid the personal suffering of the patient. Nouwen observed:

> The paradox indeed is that those who want to be for "everyone" find themselves often unable to be close to anyone. When everybody becomes my "neighbor'" it is worth wondering whether anyone really becomes my "proximus," that is, the one most close to me.[1]

To be a physician is to suffer with the patient. The guilt of physicians is that they accept the burden of providing salvation, of delivering patients from the anxiety they feel. To have skill and knowledge with which to answer the patients, using the language they use, means making a promise that is frighteningly similar to the promise of Christ, even when on a very small scale and even when so frequently misused by the patients who ask for that help. When we paraphrase Nouwen, replacing the ministry with medicine, we have the true situation:

> If there is any posture that disturbs a suffering man or woman, it is aloofness. The tragedy of [medicine] is that many who are in need, many who seek an attentive ear, a word of support, a forgiving embrace, a firm hand, a tender smile, or even a stuttering confession of inability to do more, often find that [physicians] are distant people who do not want to burn their fingers. [Physicians] are unable or unwilling to express their feelings of affection, anger, hostility or sympathy.[2]

This expected total involvement creates vulnerability in the physician. Many physicians avoid that extrapolation of their calling. They do not become mature, but stagnate in self-absorption. They still may have the virtue "care," but they will not reach wisdom.

Acknowledgment and Guilt

The specter of shouldering guilt for the patient is so frightening that physicians as a group actually warn against it. They fear over-involvement with the patient; they warn against over-identification. The quintessential Western physician is Sir William Osler. His image is still held up as the ideal for the modern medical student. In many ways, Osler typified what can be good in medicine: careful bedside observation, listening to the patient's symptoms, and interpreting of all the clues given by the patient directly, from the family, and from the social environment.

There are many Osler scholars. One of those, Dr. John P. McGovern, commented, when a medallion was struck by the American Medical Association in Osler's commemoration, as follows:

> Search as one may, throughout history there cannot be found a better example of the complete physician than William Osler. A supremely competent and dedicated clinician, renowned for his diagnostic skills, he was also, "Premier Teacher of Clinical Medicine." Additionally, he was an active investigator and discoverer in many diverse fields such as malaria, tuberculosis, and cardiovascular diseases. He published more than 1500 articles, monographs and books on a variety of medical topics, including his famous treatise on internal medicine, THE PRINCIPLES AND PRACTICE OF MEDICINE, which for fifty years, through numerous editions, served as the standard text. Osler also earned a lasting reputation as the innovator of new formats for medical education. His reforms of the medical school curriculum, which emphasizes the philosophy that the medical student should be taught clinical medicine in the wards and outpatient departments rather than just lectured to in the classroom, laid the foundation for modern medical education. He taught medical students in the wards. He also initiated the first post-doctoral intern-residency program in [the United States]. [3]

This statement is quoted from a county medical society journal. There are, of course, more scholarly publications that summarize the impact of Osler on medical education and medical practice.[4] However, the specific source quoted illustrates the continued significance of Osler for current medical practice.

The Least Among Thee

These major accomplishments in medical education alone would give Osler the place he richly deserves in American medicine. However, he is also held up as the epitome of medical humanism. To quote McGovern again:

> In the final analysis, all told Osler's greatest legacy to medicine may well have been the model he provided for his own and future students of medicine and indeed, he often said that the "message of life is greater than the message of the pen." His approach was the epitome of "holism." He found no substitute for a solid foundation in science and for hard work and thorough preparation, yet, he believed, above all else, that caring for and understanding the whole patient as a human being is the essential element in clinical medicine. He demonstrates time and again that the best in medicine emerges from that combination of scientific ability leavened with a pervasive humanism of which he was the best of examples.[5]

What Osler's life philosophy was is somewhat difficult to extract from the myths. Most physicians attribute to Osler the qualities they themselves feel make the complete physician. Medicine sometimes needs a Bultmann also.[6] But Osler did leave a personal philosophy that is so often quoted that it embodies the myth. In April 1913, Osler gave the Silliman Lecture to the undergraduates of Yale University. He called his address "A Way of Life". In that lecture he admonished the students to "live in day-tight compartments."[7] In eloquent, yet simple language, he advised:

> The load of tomorrow, added to that of yesterday, carried today makes the strongest falter. Shut off the future as tightly as the past.[8]

Of course, the concept that today is the day, get on with today's work, is real and often sound. The disciplined life is a habit. As McGovern summarized:

> Osler bade them banish the ghosts of the past, shut their minds to the specter of the future, and get on with the today's work. His theme, sounded again and again, referred to the Aristotelian concept of life as a habit and habit as the gradual acquisition of power by long practice; he entreated his audience to establish the habit of living for the day, thereby gaining mastery over body and mind.[9]

Acknowledgment and Guilt

But it is precisely the nature of illness that disease reawakens in patients the suppressed ghost of the past and conjures up the fearsome specter of a dreaded future, if not the awesome prospect of no future. If physicians are willing to share that experience with their patients, there is not enough compassion in the airtight compartment of today.

This does not imply that a physician modeled along the lines of "A Way of Life" cannot empathize with patients. Osler was fond of children and readily befriended them.[10] He was a charter member of the American Pediatric Society and encouraged participation in that new society's activities.[11] But sharing the cross of their illness does not shine through the description of Osler. Possibly, of course, the biographers merely do not want to see that challenge. The shining example of Osler, the empathic detachment of whole-body treatment of disease, may be a myth. Osler may have been more than his biographic myth-makers project. However, even in his Christian concerns, one feels a certain simplicity that keeps total commitment at arm's length:

> Begin the day with Christ and His prayer – you need no other. Creedless, with it you have religion; creed stuffed, it will leaven any theological dough in which you stick. As the soul is dyed by the thoughts, let no day pass without contact with the best literature of the world. Learn to know your Bible, though not perhaps as your fathers did. In forming character and in shaping conduct, its touch still has its ancient power.[12]

In a roundtable discussion on "The Medical Dilemma: Professional and Personal Needs," one panel member said:

> When you're in the first year of medical school, you meet some interns and residents, and they tell you about the remarkable metamorphosis that will come over you. They say that you now have unbridled, wide-eyed idealism, but in just a few years that will change to cynicism. Maybe cynicism is too harsh and pejorative a term; maybe we should say healthy skepticism. In many respects this transition does occur, and I think it is good. Maybe the ultimate model of someone with medical and personal competence

is a person who would combine the attributes of unbridled enthusiasm of a first year medical student, the omniscience and unerring judgment of a junior resident, and the perspective of the attending. At any rate, those are important qualities to be nurtured.[13]

That summarizes the Osler ideal as it is now perceived.

Another model physician is the one who avoids responsibility by avoiding a promise. Contracting with patients for their care involves risk taking. There is an implied, even though not absolute, promise of helping by curing the disease. Possibly, however, one can avoid sharing the burden by avoiding the implied promise. The paradigm for that attitude is the oncologist.[14]

Among cancer patients the quest for cure is most intense, yet the ability of the physician to deliver cure is most problematical.[15] Therefore, the motive of the physician to become an oncologist, especially a radiotherapist or chemotherapist, cannot be the satisfaction of a usually successful outcome. However, it is unlikely that it is only monetary rewards that draw oncologists to a métier that would keep physicians in a position of failure – if for no other reason that few physicians have a vulture mentality. Rather the converse: most physicians have a sincere desire to help their charges and empathize with their patients.

It is then legitimate to question what the motives of non-surgical oncologists really are. One could approach this question by an in-depth interview with a sufficient number of oncologists, but that would require time and a scope of inquiry that is hardly achievable, since such motives would not be readily discernible from just a questionnaire approach. One might also suggest that the question should be moot, since the posture of oncology should not be cure at all costs, but rather should allow supported, but minimally disturbed, dying when the disease is incurable. However, even if that attitude is granted as desirable, the fact remains that the medical profession approaches patients with, on the whole, therapeutic vigor, and that most patients initially do expect that from their doctor. That more

Acknowledgment and Guilt

physicians and patients should acknowledge the inevitable and thereby create more gracious ways of dying is without dispute. True, during the initial physician-patient contact, when the cancer is first discovered, it is possible for the patient to refuse referral to an oncologist. Whether such refusal is pragmatically impossible because of societal or familial pressure is beside the point, because such factors are outside the patient-physician contact. However, once the patient accepts the referral, the oncologist will be expected to cure, however mistaken that expectation may be.

The question is therefore legitimate: what motivates oncologists to allow them-selves to be placed in such a position? The answer could be that cancer presents the greatest remaining opportunity to alleviate human suffering, or that oncology offers the greatest remaining medical challenge, and thereby the greatest hope of personal advancement. However, it is also clear that patients with cancer are still generally expected to die, and therefore oncology offers the greatest opportunity of reward with the least danger of having to admit failure.

In these caricatures I have not spelled out the nature of rewards for the oncologist; they can range from purely selfish and monetary, through acquisition of social and academic standing, to quiet self-satisfaction. But the reward sought does not really change the oncologist's motivation.

Not all three possible motives need detailed examination. First it is clear that almost no one is motivated purely by only one of the three. Second, everyone will acknowledge that the first two motives are active to varying degrees at varying moments in most physicians. The question is really whether the third postulate – oncology is a psychologically safe field, because it is all right to fail – is indeed a possibility.

Of course, no one could live with pure and unvarying failure. The assertion that we all will die is a truism, but it is trivial and has no bearing on the physician's motivation. The goal of the oncologist is not indefinite survival; rather, the goal is that death should be from causes unrelated to cancer. But oncology is in a state of flux. Many patients *are* cured; but only in pediatric oncology, and now also in certain types of breast cancer, is cure more frequent than death. Great effort is expanded on improving those statistics. But success, during such investigational approaches, can be measured by an impact on the average course of the disease, and not necessarily by cure rate alone. In other words, significantly prolonged survival, and not necessarily cure, is accepted as a goal. This makes the posture of the oncologist potentially more secure, because reward for doing well to people, in the face of actual failure as defined by the patient, is completely possible.

What would one predict, given the notion that the physician's motive is security in expected failure and rejoicing in unexpected success. A repeated experiment actually puts this hypothesis to the test. The postulated attitude is most tenable when the projected patient outcome is as close to fifty-fifty as possible. Those chances would maximize rewards, and yet not threaten the expectation of failure because cure is the norm. Such a failure rate needs, of course, to be reduced if all patients are to be helped. Yet it is a widely observed phenomenon that if one challenges therapeutic strategies through which about 50 percent are cured, one generates opposition. The objections are that it is "unethical" to endanger the outcome of the cured to improve the outcome of the failures.

As presented here, that objection is conceptually irrational at face value. Yet, the cry of "unethical" is heard with persistent regularity, especially if one group of oncologists suggests a new mode of therapy to the proponents of the more entrenched modes of treatment. At the time of the workshop the classical confrontation occurred when it was suggested that chemotherapy replace radiotherapy: "It is unethical." That is precisely the reaction one would predict from our hypothesis.

Again, a caricature is unfair. Nevertheless, all cancer therapists should examine their motives. We do not always grieve deeply for every patient lost, because we know our limitations; we cannot morbidly grieve for the inevitable as long as we know we have done our best and not made inadvertent or careless errors. The problem is not that this attitude is wrong, but that we are at ease with that attitude.

During a workshop in our department of pediatrics it was very evident that the concept of cure is threatening.[16] All oncologists are, to a degree, ambivalent, and the hypothesis that we are at ease with not having to account for failure fits the observed behavioral facts uncomfortably well. Many physicians say they could not do what oncologists are doing. Yet in no field are the rewards greater. Oncologists do not deal with a patient population of which more than 80 percent get better in spite of the physician, as the primary practitioner does. Therefore the few cures can be claimed as personal accomplishment far more often in oncology than in any other branch of medicine where cures are possible. That, indeed, is stimulus but the security may be that failure is not always threatening.

At the present time, this motive serves the oncologist as well as any, because non-cure is still so overwhelmingly the norm that treatment improvements can be sought actively by all oncologists without changing the conceptual view of cancer as a deadly disease. Very few patients suffer as a result of the physician's attitude; indeed, care is optimal because, inherent in the non-threat of failure, remains the needed conviction of having delivered optimal care. But oncology is making great strides and, it is hoped, a new generation of oncologists will take over who will view the care of cancer patients with motives more in harmony with the patient's expectations. It is even possible, if not likely, that oncology will become a routine branch of primary care medicine. Then our current conceptual equating cancer with death and unpleasant dying will no longer be possible. The special motives of oncologists need no longer be postulated.

Another way in which the physician can avoid maturity, and thereby avoid shouldering of the burden of the patient, is by assuming total control. The need to fight death at every last drawn battle line can be so overwhelming that one gives little thought to the consequences that the patient suffers from being that battlefield. Bartholome's concern has already been cited.[17] The reality of experiencing cancer is where the most fear of annihilation, loneliness and hopelessness is found in patients.

In spite of all our current discussions about brain death, the vast majority of people still conceive the heart as the measure of life – not necessarily as the seat of the soul, and therefore not as the equivalent of the person, but rather as the index of life in the body, which is the vessel of the spirit. Therefore the threat to the heart is seen as an all or none threat. If the heart fails, then the body is gone, and the spirit may even be thought of as liberated. If there is any image of resurrection, fears are allayed since the body is still very much intact, and only a failing heart has to be restored.

Cancer, in contrast to heart disease, is far more likely to encroach on far less vital parts. The progressive destruction of the body without a concomitant liberation of the spirit is to many very frightening. Eventually death may occur, and the body seems to be destroyed with a heart that is still viable. To be able to incorporate any concept of immortality requires far greater power of imagination and rationalization under such circumstances. Even though the separation of body and spirit is widely discussed and mostly acknowledged, the conceptualization of being dead, if it is forced upon one at all, very much involves living images. A brain death is very frightening, because it conjures up an image of a spirit that could not escape the body in time to wait for reclamation of that body. To most people a brain death is only conceivable in others. Cancer death is seen as the converse: no real workable body for the spirit to survive in, but a spirit that has not yet been liberated. And brain tumors are the most feared of all.[18]

To share that burden of annihilation as the cross our patients challenge us to endure is so frightening that physicians feel that the disease does indeed need to be fought at all hazards. As one medical oncologist once said:

> The physician is often called upon to serve patients whose lives will be shortened by their illness. The physician is repeatedly called upon to assist

his patient to face the inevitability of death. Many proponents of "death with dignity" raise the illusion of the patient in his bed at home in a stately pose, with bright, clean, freshly pressed sheets, in a lovely room with a warm fire in the fireplace, surrounded by his friends, associates and family, whispering his final words before he turns his head to the side and closes his eyes forever. As physicians we know that this is an illusion. Death is almost invariably a horrible event. The things that accompany dying include convulsions, emesis, involuntary diarrhea, hemorrhage with blood on all the surrounding surfaces, involuntary shrieks, pain, suffering, dehydration, anorexia, etc. The ugliness and horror of dying are experiences that physicians live with daily; lay people cannot anticipate this ugliness. The cry for an individual to die at home is completely contradictory to human experience.[19]

With that kind of an attitude, that physician has to fight death as an enemy. Dying is not a meaningful experience, and the threat of dying is not a suffering to be shared. Freireich elaborates:

In my view, death is always ugly, undesirable, and the ultimate enemy of man. It is the physician's responsibility to assist the patient in facing fatal illness with COURAGE. To supplement that outrage with relief of suffering using whatever intellectual, emotional, and physical support he can muster is the socially vital role that the physician offers to each individual who voluntarily elects to become a patient. The physician needs no defense. He has, throughout recorded history of the human species, been one of the most essential professional members of every human community. For it is the physician, through his professional competence, who relieves suffering and prolongs life. We should not veer from that essential role.[20]

If the battle seems lost, there must have been a flaw in the strategy: research therapy must be resorted to. Such a physician takes literally the language the physical disease uses to convey the ontological threat, just as a deaf person often gives a very literal interpretation of the meaning of words. For the deaf, in their ponderous process of mastering any language at all, there is no way to learn the "meaning of meaning."[21] Their grammar is simplistic; for them to perceive the basis of transformational grammar is nearly impossible.[22]

The Least Among Thee

The analogy is serious. The physician can have a deaf ear to the patient. This deafness results in simple interpretation of the language used by the patient. The interpretation becomes very literal indeed.

In order to wage that all-out battle, the physician must control the patient totally. On occasion the guilt of failure is then transferred to the patient. The patient, or the disease, did not allow the cure. One should not get the impression that physicians with this attitude are simplistic persons, rather the converse. They are enormously complex persons, who must fight off the overpowering call for help of patients. Freireich has said elsewhere:

> Nor should a physician ever play the role of judge. It is incorrect and improper for a physician in his professional role to try to make judgments about whether or not a patient is suffering. Although we all think it is relatively simple to determine when someone is suffering, it is not, in actuality, an easy thing to do.[23]

He places the burden of communication entirely on the patient:

> If a physician has humility and respect for life and if he is willing to admit that his own personal perspective of what's going on in a patient's mind depends entirely on that person's ability to communicate it, then I think concepts like terminal illness take on a different perspective. I don't think there is any such thing as a terminal case. The concept of "terminal" is subjective. From the moment of conception until death we are all terminal cases. We all know how it's going to come out. But we also hope that, if we become ill, there will be a good doctor around.[24]

But communication requires a receiver as well as a sender. A person can communicate effectively only when a listener understands perfectly. To try to understand one's patient perfectly requires sharing the suffering – not just hearing it, not just empathizing with it, but sharing it in all its horror.

To be a physician who is able to live in airtight compartments of the now means to care, but also to be more involved with self-absorption than

74

with generativity. The old Erikson term "stagnation" applies even better. Adulthood cannot proceed smoothly to maturity. Assuming total control is analogous to guarding against over-involvement, but is best described as self-absorption. Selecting a medical model wherein it is all right to fail is avoiding the integrity of maturity and ultimately giving in to despair. "Care" is then a virtue acquired and exercised, but "wisdom" is not.

When one takes on the care of the dying patient, a promise of healing is implied. The patient sees the cure as the way of avoiding self-annihilation. It is thought cure restores old ways. That is, of course, not so. But the patient does request the cure, and the healing that is promised initially implies that such a cure can be given. When a patient gradually sees the reality of dying, the physician has assumed the guilt of not fulfilling the promise.

Many patients are terminally ill in the sense that no known cure can be extracted of the tired body in which they live. But to call those patients dying before they call themselves dying is psychological euthanasia.

We are so often preoccupied with the quality of life. Because physicians frequently feel that the quality of a patient's life may be inferior, they are more often perturbed by last-ditch efforts than they are by peaceful death. Physicians often prepare patients for their demise. After all, it is easier to tolerate dying as the norm and reap the occasional cure as a reward than it is to expect cure and accept death as failure. Physicians have, by this attitude, allowed themselves the luxury of euthanasia. This psychological euthanasia, however, is no better than physical euthanasia. Telling patients prematurely they are going to die becomes a self-fulfilling prophesy. That does not mean that telling the truth is not desirable, but the truth must be objective, and the motives behind rushing the death prediction are often far removed from those engendered by objectivity.[25]

There is only one person who can say that he or she is dying, and that is the patient. Only when that realization is incorporated into living is it a reality. Until a patient wants to acknowledge dying, the realization of the imminence of death is so profoundly frightening to the patient as to be unacceptable. That burden is carried for the patient by the physician. Brody, in a short editorial on hope in medical care[26], quoted Emily Dickinson:

> The heart asks pleasure first –
> and then – escape from pain –
> and then – those little anodynes
> that deaden suffering –
>
> and then – to go to sleep –
> and then – if it should be
> the will of its inquisitor –
> the privilege to die.[27]

Through a slow progression the patient handles the approaching self-dissolution. The physician who is asked to stop the progression may well know the inability to do so, but carries that load for the patient.

There is profound suffering in being a physician to a patient who may die. We learn that no human interaction is possible without involvement. The physician is not just a mechanic, and cannot be an unbiased observer of other people: mere presence alters the life of the one observed. Even just befriending is traumatic. Befriending is involvement with another person, and only when we are involved are we available. We cannot use anger as a releasing emotion when losing a friend; only sadness remains.

When the reason for befriending the sick stranger is the skill one possesses as a physician, then the befriending demands more than availability; it demands that we carry the burden. It demands being the Good Samaritan over and over again. It is indeed seeing the call of God to the patient, and in turn being called by the patient to intercede. In a sense, one carries the illness and all its implications to God for absolution of the patient.

That attitude toward being a physician is one against which rebellion almost certainly occurs. But when one accepts the calling, then all debates about telling the truth, about obtaining consent, are won. One tells the patient how one is going to carry the burden, how the disease must be handled to remove the illness in the total man. Of course one tells the truth. To lie would be to destroy the help. Lipkin, in a lay press article in *Newsweek*, defended lying to patients, because it is usually a practical impossibility to tell the whole truth. He actually argued that, often enough, the ethics of the situation, the true moral responsibility, may demand that the observed fact not be revealed. He suggested that the crucial question is whether the deception was intended to benefit the patient or the doctor.[28] However, the same can be said for telling the truth.[29] The crucial question is whether the *truth* is intended to benefit the patient or the doctor. Neither telling the harsh truth nor hiding the ugly facts helps the patient if it is done to manipulate the patient into a preconceived state of optimal mental peace.

Brody said correctly that "hope is not automatically equated with survival." [30] But what, indeed, do patients hope for? Ultimately patients hope to feel whole, to be healed. A physician who becomes such a great factor in the life of the patient becomes the mediator of that hope. Patients really do not expect certainty. In fact, certainty is a very poor substitute for hope. But to be the object of the call and question voiced in the psalms is very difficult.

> And now Lord, for what do I wait?
> My hope is with thee ... [31]

We are ill-prepared to carry other people's crosses. To say that one is willing to take on another's suffering is only so much bravura – only one person did that, and He did that once and for all.

And yet, the observation is true that "In the practice of our art it often matters little what medicine is given, but it matters much that we give ourselves with our pills." [32] A profound guilt is generated by the conflict between the demand to follow Christ's example of shouldering other people's burdens in order that they may live, and the knowledge that such self-sacrifice simply cannot be made.

The Least Among Thee

Each patient views impending death so differently that there is no one way to be learned so that we might help all sufferers. When gifted writers describe their experience with an illness that they perceive as a threat to their being, very different works result. Cousins relates his feeling of helplessness in the hospital, his fear of never returning to normalcy, his fear of being thought a complainer. His conflict was between the terror of loneliness and the desire to be left alone. An utter void was created by the longing – ineradicable, unremitting, pervasive – for the warmth of human contact.[33] Malreaux, on the other hand, told us: "I am disconcerted by the absence of pain. Death, in our minds, is so powerfully linked with pain that we are stunned by an illness which may be mortal but which does not torture us – dumbfounded by the most disconcerting divorce of our time." [34]

There is still fear in having to respond to that call for help in all its varied and anxious tones. Many physicians hope that there are subsets of medicine that are inherently more responsive to the cries and therefore in themselves will constitute an answer to the cry for help. Family medicine declined steadily in the first half of the twentieth century,[35] but recently the number of training programs in family medicine has markedly increased. However, the challenges of the community soon frustrate. The system, even the system of family practice, cannot allow an individual to set the exclusive tone. The unique patient-doctor encounter must eventually be individualized.[36] Reliance on a system will eventually produce the despair of Sisyphus in the physician. It is true that both Sisyphus and Prometheus were condemned because the displeased the gods, but Sisyphus was dishonest and Prometheus tried to do good. They could be an analogy in the choice between the individual approaches in public and family health care.[37] However, the individual physicians who rely on the good of the institution in which they are practicing cannot reach independent integrity and wisdom. The struggle eventually generates despair, and the approach to family practice becomes as much a science as is any specialty.[38] Family practice generates a skill that allows a patient-physician encounter no more and no less than a super-specialty.

Acknowledgment and Guilt

It is true that family practice takes place in an environment that is more familiar, and therefore may be less (and occasionally more) forbidding than a remote hospital. But a patient does not have to be a number in a big institution. Patients have names and all health-care providers can use that name if the patient states it. How far health care providers will go in carrying the patient's burden is independent of the setting. Sometimes, in a hospital, it is a little easier for a physician to hide behind the various masks available – professional language, cynicism, materiality, impersonality, ritualized action, and hospital routine.[39] But that busy environment also generates an opportunity to feel for the plight of the patient. The feelings of Norman Cousins are those shared by almost all patients in a big medical center. They are frightened alone, which should therefore make hearing their threatened feelings even easier.

Physicians are called to heal, to shoulder the suffering. There will be times when it is all too much, when memories of promises we are unable to keep tumble down in the mind, even though we try eternally to rearrange them to be less threatening. But carry the load we are called to do, without the power of a God who can freely forgive others.

Physicians have the skills to lighten burdens, to allow a patient to ease into reality, to integrate past experiences. Memories are what shape us. Nouwen correctly stated,

> "Our memory plays a central role in our sense of being. Our pains and joys, our feelings of grief and satisfaction, are not simply dependent on the events of our lives, but also, and even more so, on the ways we remember these events."[40]

We have enough to carry from our own past. We cannot easily be burdened with other people's burdens, especially when they are so ontologically laden as those of the dying patient. We cannot really integrate such grating pain, because we have no reference to it other than our open and unrestrained humanity. And yet, we take the burden and lighten the load for our overburdened patients. We acquire the guilt and the need for forgiveness.

We physicians sin by usurping the power to forgive; we are pressed into sanctity by the miraculous healing we are asked to perform. There still is a lot of priesthood in medicine: it is indeed the last helping profession. Religion today offers so little promise when disease strikes, because physicians, not priests, are seen as the mediators of help. Two thousand years ago pilgrims went to the Asclepeion at Epidaurus, to be healed of their disease. They received massages, baths, and the psychotherapy of faith. Today, physicians are the chosen mediators. Physicians promise. They do not always deliver. They are guilty of being imperfect priests. Our patients challenge us continually. One of our mental health workers quoted a poem by Medina:

> If this is not a place where tears are understood,
>   Where do I go to cry?
> If this is not a place where my spirits can take wing,
>   Where do I go to fly?
> If this is not a place where my questions can be asked,
>   Where do I go to seek?
> If this is not a place where my feelings can be heard,
>   Where do I go to speak?
> If this is not a place where you'll accept me as I am,
>   Where can I go to be?
> If this is not a place where I can try and learn, and grow,
>   Where can I just be me?
> If this is not a place where tears are understood,
>   Where can I go to cry? [41]

We take on that load by creating such a place for the burdened patient. We understand tears, allow questions. By helping to hold the burden for a moment, we allow spirits to soar at times of crushing loads. All the anxieties expressed by the patient, who says, "I am sick, help me," are ours. The burden is enormous.

Acknowledgment and Guilt

I still hear one of my fellows say:

> It is often difficult for us to convey our concerns for families and children under our care because of social precedents and personal concerns. How does one replenish the drawn energies of shared setbacks in a profession that consumes reserves? How can I genuinely care for my patients and stand back and be a calloused director of their care at the same time? Where do I go to cry or to mourn the loss of a friend? [42]

The moment comes when we are helpless beneath this crushing burden. Yet we must maintain the integrity of the patient. We may, indeed, become emotionally depleted. As physicians, we may be tempted to take over, to create dependency on the part of the patient, but that is not helpful. That does not allow patients to hand over their burden. When Christ died for our sins, he did so without destroying our freedom. We are free to believe. We are free to use Him; we are free to feel forgiven. The patient deserves no less from us. We cannot heal and control at the same time. We must allow autonomy.

We will, without fail, become wounded healers. We will carry the burden of God's children. As physicians, we are, indeed, the chosen, and we allowed ourselves to be chosen. But the burden of the chosen is as heavy as the burden of the rejected.

But how could we do otherwise? How can we avoid the cry for help; how can we turn a deaf ear? When we have the strength to help, and the skills and means to allow help to be given, we cannot, in the eyes of God, fail to give it. And yet we are destined to fail, as often as not, because in helping we take on God. We are guilty in failure and in success.

All saints of the church profess to be the greatest sinners, not because their transgressions are greater on an absolute scale, but because they are greater on the relative scale of their sanctity. Physicians can shoulder burdens as human to human, but as saints they know and accept the burden because they may understand what it is.

The Least Among Thee

Such a burden cannot be carried alone. The accumulated guilt must be atoned for. We cannot live without help.

> How long, O Lord, wilt thou quite forget me?
> How long wilt thou hide thy face from me?
> How long must I suffer anguish in my soul,
> grief in my heart, day and night?
> How long shall my enemy lord over me?
> Look now and answer me, O Lord my God.
> Give light to my eyes lest I sleep the sleep of death,
> lest my adversary say: 'I have overthrown him,'
> and my enemies rejoice at my downfall.[43]

It is possible to try to protect oneself from despair by drawing a line on the continuum of involvement and non-involvement. One can argue that over-involvement and over-identification can limit the physician's ability to exercise rational thinking,[44] but this argument does not help despair. In the rock opera *Jesus Christ Superstar*, there is a scene in the Temple where Christ is crowded by all the sick, the lame, the poor, in a crescendo of supplicating horror, until he cries out:

> So many of you –
> Too little of me –
> Don't crowd me –
> Heal thyself, …

And he is soothed by temptation when Mary Magdalene sings:

> Try not to get worried,
> try not to turn onto
> problems that upset you;
> don't you know everything's
> alright, everything's fine?
> Close your eyes, close your eyes
> and forget all about us tonight.[45]

Acknowledgment and Guilt

But it was not possible for Jesus to be satisfied with that, nor is it possible for us. We must provide help, and we must also seek help ourselves. We are called to help and we are stripped naked and drained spiritually. We cannot say, "Go away and heal thyself," because we know they know not how. We begin to call for help ourselves:

> Answer me when I call, O God, maintainer of my right,
> I was hard pressed, and thou didst set me at large,
> Be gracious to me now and hear my prayer.[46]

We can only reach that point if there is little lingering doubt – if we truly understand what our calling is, and what the burden is that we shoulder.

The mass begins with the *Kyrie*: "Lord, have mercy upon me."

De profundo clamavi ad te.[47]

CHAPTER V

Atonement

Atonement

To be a true helper without overwhelming the helped leaves one lonely and wounded. Help is needed for the physician also. The help is not truly available from within ourselves. What the physician needs is to be forgiven for the accumulated guilt. There has to be atonement. It is too empty within ourselves.

> And lonely as it is, that loneliness
> will be more lonely ere it will be less,
> a blanket whiteness of brightened snow
> with no expression, nothing to express.
> They cannot scare me with their empty spaces
> between stars – on stars where no human race is.
> I have it in me so much nearer home
> to scare myself with my own desert places.[1]

But to be forgiven requires acknowledgment of guilt. One cannot obtain atonement without confession. First are the sins we commit ourselves, as human beings. And for a physician, there are the greater sins of promising salvation and not delivering it, or of helping and thereby thwarting God. Physicians, in answering their calling, enter a serving profession that demands action *in loco Jesu*. We take on God by speaking for Him. That challenge is real and is our task. But unless we are willing to acknowledge our sins – sins that we are called to make, that our calling forced upon us – we cannot be forgiven.

The Least Among Thee

Sometimes others who have thought long and hard about a phrase say it better than we can ourselves. The language of the bishops of Vatican II is clear, explicit and direct:

> The Lord Jesus, divine teacher and model of all perfection, preached holiness of life (of which he is the author and maker) to each and every one of his disciples without distinction: "You, therefore, must be perfect, as your heavenly father is perfect.[2]

That is a general challenge and admonition. But the physician sees a special meaning in that calling.

The temptation certainly exists to remain isolated in our darkness. There is a soothing beauty in our isolation – to give up, to let it all become quiet, white, and covered, to stand still and forget. See and feel, again, the imagery of Robert Frost:

> Whose woods these are I think I know.
> His house is in the village though;
> He will not see me stopping here
> To watch his woods fill up with snow.
>
> My little horse may think it queer
> To stop without a farmhouse near
> Between the woods and frozen lake
> The darkest evening of the year.
>
> He gives his harness bells a shake
> To ask if there is some mistake.
> The only other sound's the sweep
> Of easy wind and downy flake.
>
> The woods are lovely, dark and deep,
> But I have promises to keep,
> And miles to go before I sleep
> And miles to go before I sleep.[3]

Atonement

The woods are a lovely temptress, who is both immediate life and prolonged death. And yet we do have promises to keep. Sleep and deliverance may be a long way off.

To give up can become an overwhelming temptation. We often hear descriptions of the drowning victim who feels drawn to the release of giving up. The feeling of release – that allows one not to struggle anymore. Today the release through giving up has become almost codified. We call it "burnout," and we hold seminars on how to prevent it from happening or how to give in to burnout because one is truly not suitable to the profession. Of course, that can be the case. But giving in to burnout is also declaring a spiritual bankruptcy that can only be acceptable in a value system that avoids commitment. We make temptation so easy to give in to, and we make avoiding the difficult so acceptable, that difficulty ceases to have inherent virtue.

The temptation not to go on, not to load more guilt upon oneself, becomes more powerful the heavier the load is. The snow covers all the rough ground that needs to be covered. The grounds are lovely, as is a woman who promises rest in mystery. We hear the twinkle of the bells on the horse, but even that sound belongs to the snowy woods – conscience can be interpreted so differently depending on when we hear its voice. Ultimately, however, the promise the physicians have to keep makes them go onward, knowing full well they still have a long road ahead before they will hear, "Well done, thou good and faithful servant." [4]

> But I have promises to keep,
> And miles to go before I sleep.

There is a real analogy between the physician and the priest. Nouwen's observations about the minister fit the physician totally. Both physicians and ministers may often want to run away to hide and play deaf, dumb, and blind for a while. But because we are physicians, we must, by listening, heal the wounds of the past; by our skill, sustain life in the present; and by our guidance, steer our patients into the future. All the dying and living people remind us again and again, "And so we keep returning to our vocation and growing strong in humility and love." [5]

But in so doing we utterly and completely humiliate ourselves in the knowledge of our guilt. To acknowledge the Christian faith and claim forgiveness is not sufficient. In addition we must confess our unworthiness, our inability to respond to our patients' call for omnipotence – an omnipotence that we know we do not possess. All saints of the church have had to make this two-step acknowledgment of the salvation of Christ. Belief, and the total faith required to survive, requires total understanding of one's fallibility. When we discover ourselves as we are, we discover Christ as He is.

Physicians promise more than most humans, and, therefore, need Christ all the more. But in Christ lies the power and strength to go on. So many others have discovered that universal truth, not just physicians. We listen to those who have been through this experience and say, "Yes – yes that is it; that is the way it is."

> True encounter with Christ
> liberates something in us,
> a power we did not know we had,
> a hope, a capacity for life,
> a resilience, an ability to bounce back
> when we thought we were completely defeated.[6]

If we truly admit our fallibility, if we freely accept our patients' burdens and let them be freed of their fears, then indeed Christ will know us. We are freed from our sins because of Christ's sacrifice, because of the cross. We must understand that our actions for our patients demand our sacrifice for them. Only then are we worthy of the salvation of Christ's sacrifice. But when we go from being our patients' neighbor to sacrificing ourselves for them, in order to be worthy of our Lord's sacrifice and thereby to be relieved of guilt, we no longer feel that sacrifice is something subjective and hard.

Atonement

Sacrifice is something objective. It is a deliberate act, a knowing serving. It is not difficult or painful when we do it for the glory of God. Only when we rebel, only when our weakness makes us shy away from the challenge so that we are in conflict with God, does sacrifice become difficult. The difficulty then ensues only from our conflict with God, not from the burden of the task. The perfect sacrifice should be painless: "a pure act of adoration, a hymn to the divine glory sung in ecstatic peace." [7] That divine peace comes from being the mediator of Christ's salvation to our patients. Our intervention is the intervention of the Lord.

And yet, acknowledging that blessed relief from our guilt, realizing our salvation, often makes us rear up and assert our assumed power all the more. We want to control that new power. We want to show our miraculous powers. Does the Bible not say, "Ask, and you will receive; seek, and you will find; knock, and the door will be opened." [8] We demand the power to heal. We forget the context Jesus established later: "Get your mind on God's kingdom and his justice before everything else, and all the rest will come to you as well." [9]

The desire to take on the power to undo the evil in the world is dormant in all of us. When, as physicians, we have a small touch of the power, we want not only to use it as God directs but also to use it because we think we know best. This demand for power because of our imagined, all-envisioning wisdom is a new temptation on the road to peace. [10] We are so frequently like the sorcerer's apprentice, playing with power we cannot control.

When we know God to be merciful, when we know our faith can allow us truly to supplicate and be heard, we want even more. The more we learn the power of God's faith in us, the more we learn to understand the sorrow and misery of all humans. We hear them all around us, we see them every day, we read about them around the world. When I care for a child with cancer and try to support his or her anguished parents, I cannot help but question the need for all that suffering. By giving hope, by alleviating pain, by fighting the disease, we can help; we can make that suffering a little less. By helping the family to understand that it is normal to have cancer, even for a child, we help carry the burden. When God then allows us to succeed in curing, when our skills are in fact sufficient, we understand for a fleeting moment the mercy of God.

I remember one time I saw a child look at me asking to please leave me alone, to please let him have the liberation of death. Then I agonized with the parents and grandparents, who tried so hard to help their eldest son. They were God-fearing parents who saw in me the physical evidence of the power of God, who was going to show His justice after all. But Sammy will die, perhaps not immediately, but soon. In the parents there is hope that maybe death is best for Sammy. The parents show their humanity in both their search for the best for Sammy, and in their fear of loss. When, as a physician, I can slowly affect healing in the parents, I know that God grants me power. When that healing power belongs not just to me, but also to an entire therapeutic community that understands, supports, listens, cries, and laughs with the parents and Sammy, then I know that God will let us make a better world than we have.

> If we die with him, we shall live with him;
> If we endure, we shall reign with him;
> If we deny him, he will deny us.
> If we are faithless, he keeps faith,
> for he cannot deny himself.[11]

It is said that God created us little lower than the angels; but that applies to all men, not just physicians. Our skills make us have a special calling, but not a superior position in the hierarchy. Our patients are not creatures of God over which physicians have been made master. [12] We must wait for the cry for help to come to us; we should not presume to answer cries not voiced but only imagined, to show our special relationship to God. This is a temptation that we need to reject as certainly as the temptation of giving up, of losing ourselves in the lovely, deep, dark woods of helplessness.

Atonement

To allow God to act through us requires a self-negation that will create constant pressure. To be the conduit of God's compassion for the patient under our care is indeed to become acquainted with all the misery of the human, but also to know all the counterbalancing goodness of a forgiving God. It is not in our patients that the battle is fought, but in us. We need help ourselves. We need to call on God for help, as well as for power to heal, and the call for help must come first. We must learn that we are alone and the handler of the fear for the patient. We must call for an answer:

> How long, O Lord wilt thou quite forget me?
> How long wilt thou hide thy face from me?
> How long must I suffer anguish in my soul,
> grief in my heart day and night? [13]

And that same psalm gives the answer:

> But for my part I trust in thy true love.
> My heart shall rejoice, for thou hast set me free.
> I will sing to the Lord, who has granted all my desires.[14]

Our desire is help for the patient. But the more we are open to the misery of the patient, the more help we need ourselves. The more the patients let us know what this disease means for them, and the more their fears of self-annihilation show through, the more we need strength to make our skills work. When we can acknowledge that we ourselves must cry for help, when we can feel the need, eventually we can call:

> My God, my God, why hast thou forsaken me
> and art so far from saving me, from heeding my groans? [15]

When we call on God like that, help is most fully at hand. Then we can die for our patients, to be reawakened in Christ. Once we have called like that we know the answer comes; we feel the true peace of faith, in fact, a joy of giving that can only be seen in those who are at ease with their own inadequacy. There is great joy in being able to use a skill to help, however inadequate it is. There is great joy in being able to heal, in being called to do so because one is a physician and allowed to do so because one is willing to become the locus of battle between misery and grace.

The first time we have overcome the temptation to give up, and we have also overcome the temptation to usurp power not granted, we will have to fight off the temptation to evangelize instead of to heal. We do not need to proclaim our sanctity to our patients. We are not called to become evangelizing preachers for their salvation.

It is not the power of the word, nor the power of the conviction, that proves our liberation from guilt. Rather, once we truly feel liberated, freedom ceases to be an issue. It is the way we are. Freedom cannot be taught; it can only be lived. It cannot be preached, but only shown. If we truly believe we cannot help ourselves, we must do – we are powerfully ordained to do – what the patient needs. We are healers of illness. That is our challenge; that is the wording of the supplication by the patient to God.

To be a Christian physician is to be a Christian and to be a physician. There is no need to proclaim the faith; such proclamation is likely to be directed at ourselves rather than at the patient. Remember the apostle James, who said:

> What use is it for a man to say he has faith when he does nothing to show it? Can that faith save him? Suppose a brother or a sister is in rags with not enough food for the day, and one of you says, "Good luck to you, keep yourselves warm, and have plenty to eat, but does nothing to supply their bodily needs, what is the good of that? So with faith, if it does not lead to action, it is itself a lifeless thing. But someone may object: 'Here is one who claims to have faith and another who points to his deeds.' To which I reply: 'Prove to me that this faith you speak of is real though not accompanied by deeds and by my deeds I will prove to you may faith.' You have faith enough to believe there is one God. Excellent. The devils have faith like that, and it makes them tremble. But can you not see, you quibbler, that faith divorced from deeds is barren? [16]

Atonement

There is no need to convince anyone. There is no need to complain. The patient asks for help through the illness, and we act through the illness. We heal by God's grace, through our deeds and in His name. We get no credit for succeeding and we receive forgiveness for failing.

Only with that conviction can we accept that there really is no failure in our unfulfilled promise. This is not because we are limited in our capabilities and cannot truly promise, but we can indeed help because there is no failure in the patient who dies. Death is a failure of our human promise, which was our human answer to our patient's human request. But when our actions are more than human – when they are the expression of our faith – we see that death is as much a promise as life, and that God's action through us may liberate from fear in many ways. Espousing either the will to live or the wish to die can resolve the dilemma posed by the life-threatening illness. Which resolution is God's will, we cannot presume to know. We can only hope, as physicians, to alleviate suffering, to help reduce the impact of the disease, and to continue to listen to the patient for the message that is conveyed.

Death is not always the enemy. It is not even the target of the concern about the illness. It is the concern itself. We cannot resolve the patient's dilemma by using death to alleviate suffering. The physical pain, the burden of illness, is our legitimate target, the one against which all our skills must be brought to bear. But to use euthanasia as the solution is doubly wrong. It avoids sharing the suffering, and it forces a solution from pain where the pain was seen as the metaphor for the death. It is like breaking a mirror for someone who did not like her looks.

There is another reason why death may not be used to treat a physical illness. The ultimate discourtesy to God is to appear before Him before we are summoned. To hasten death would be to insult God. However, death can be to ourt patients either a frightening enemy or a longed-for friend. We must come to understand that death may also be a friend and an ally for us when we are healing in the name of God. Whenever death is identified

95

as the enemy of the physician, as the target of our counter-attack, I quote the stanza by Swinburne:

> From too much love of living, from hope and fear set free,
> We thank with brief thanksgiving whatever gods may be,
> That no life lives forever;
> That dead men rise up never;
> That even the weariest river winds somewhere safe to sea. [17]

Death can be rest for the patient. Death is the resolution of the patients' anxiety. When a patient is dying, when the patient accepts the imminence of death, our tasks becomes harder. Then we stand by, help, support, understand – and let the last struggle be fought in our minds. Our decisions must be made to help and not to hinder, without making death come before the patients is ready to receive death. We must continue to decide in the name of the Lord. The agony of decision must be ours alone; we cannot transfer that burden to the patient.

Ours is an age that emphasizes informed consent. There are as many proponents who insist that a fully informed patient is the only freely deciding patient as there are opponents who insist that a truly informed patient is impossible.

Both views are completely correct. The central concern, however, is the courtesy of freedom that we must extend to our patients. They must be allowed to decide for themselves, but they must not be forced to make decisions in order that the doctor can avoid a decision. The concept of informed consent assumes that "yes" and "no" are equally acceptable answers. The agony of determining what to decide about, remains the physicians'. The physician must first be convinced that the alternatives offered are the best ones available.

At present, our medical establishment has generally available a number of mechanisms for research therapy. Therefore, physicians must be very clear what they are offering to the patient. Major difficulties and conflicts have arisen in this area. For instance, as I have written elsewhere:

> … since more than half of all children with cancer are now referred to tertiary institutions where clinical trials are being conducted, the trial has become the accepted mode of therapy. In fact, enrollment in protocols is often continued when no new protocol is available because oncologists have no alternative. Institutional Review Boards[18] are continually shamed into hastily approving chemotherapeutic experiments because there are patients who are said to need the drug, or who would otherwise die quickly. It is clear that there is no clear concept of experiment left in may of our current generation of pediatric (and adult) oncologists. If we know a drug is effective, no experiment is needed; if we really do not know, careful consideration and meaningful participation by the patient are essential. Dying patients do not benefit from the conceptual confusion of their physicians.[19]

The content of the research is the basic ethical question. Once that is answered, then informed content is possible for the patient. The struggle for the physician is all the greater in that setting.

We are captive of our role, and precisely because we are such captives we have hope of salvation and liberation. Precisely because of the difficult task of our self-negating care is our hope maximized. Karl Barth preached from time to time in the prison of Basel, Switzerland, while he was professor of theology at Basel University. In theological circles, the age of Barth has mostly past, but Barth had an enormous impact on the post World War II renewal of the confessional church. His insistence on the credo and his elaboration of dogma offered individuals a renewed interest in theology that was sorely needed at the time. Barth knew that God is exalted and man is lost in sin, but also that salvation is the ultimate gracious act of God. Barth preached to the prisoners, because they were an understandable metaphor of all humanity's condition. He preached to prisoners and thereby preached to himself.

The Least Among Thee

The physician is in an analogous situation to the prisoner: the state of being a physician is, in a way, also an acute metaphor of all humanity. Therefore, the prayers of Barth in prison, for prisoners, become poignant prayers for physicians:

> We spread before thee all that troubles us, our mistakes, our errors and our transgressions, our sorrows and cares, also our rebellion and our bitterness – our whole heart, our whole life, better known to thee than it is to ourselves. We commit all this into the faithful hands, which thou has outstretched in our Savior. Take us as we are; strengthen us when we are weak; grant us, the poor, the bounties of thy blessing.[20]

When we become truly convinced of the promise of God's salvation, we face the ultimate temptation. Total self-negation is given to very few among us, and then only to those chosen who, indeed, can concentrate on God. But the physician who has followed the path the calling indicates, and who has become a mature adult, will see glimpses of God's almighty grace. Thos glimpses can bring forth an unquenchable longing, a desire to partake more and more of that grace. To follow that vision requires a self-negation beyond anything that can be humanly maintained while yet participating in society.

The consuming mysticism of Saint John of the Cross contains profound truths. His famous poem, central to his way must be understood before such a vision of total concentration on God could be realized:

> If you want to have pleasure in everything,
>   You must desire to have pleasure in nothing.
>
> If you want to possess everything,
>   You must desire to have nothing.
>
> If you want to become all
>   You must desire to be nothing.

Atonement

If you want to know all,
  You must desire to know nothing.

If you want to arrive at that which you know not,
  You must go by a way which you know not.

If you want to arrive at that which you possess not,
  You must go by a way which you possess not.

If you want to arrive at that which you are not,
  You must pass through that which you are not.[21]

But when one pursues that path to its logical end, to its all-consuming union with the All, one becomes contemplative, wholly dedicated to God, wholly turned to God. It is likely that such a saint could heal by his very presence. There would be no impedance to the flow of divine mercy. But such healing would not be an exercise of acquired skill. There would be no person to whom the patient could relate: all cures would become miraculous. There would only be Lourdes and no hospitals.

We shy away from such profound self-abnegation. We say we do not understand it. We find counter-reformation mysticism beyond our value system. And yet, in fact, we all profoundly aspire to that peace, even as we fear the strenuous demands the ascent to Mount Carmel makes. While we may not embark on that journey, our longing for that all-consuming peace can be the last temptation of the believing physician.

However, such sanctity would not allow us to be physicians. It is precisely in our humanity that our healing power lies. We are conduits.

Physicians are humans with special skills and special calling. We must take on the burden of that humanity that makes our action as mediators of healing the burden of our God-given free choice. We are to act as free in God's name as our patient is free to receive or reject our advice.

The Least Among Thee

Yet it is not enough to be human:

> It is not then enough that men, who give
> The best gifts of man to man, should feel
> Alive, a snake's head ever at their heel.[22]

We must realize that we act *in loco Jesu*. We are forgiven, but not one time for all future transgressions. The snake's head is ever at our heel, we can be poisoned by our very humanity. Our knowledge can become the snake's bite. We need to take on God, and yet try to do His will again and again. We have the burden of choice again and again. Yet we can feel forgiven again and again. We become crucified again and again and are resurrected each time. "We are cast into that deadly silent inconceivability which radiates loneliness and which Christians call 'the cross.'"[23] We can only bear it, ask forgiveness for imitating Christ in that manner, and press on.

We do have the language of sickness to mediate the healing. When God heals, He uses our hands to do so. We translate the infinitely profound language of healing into the crude sign language of our helping hands. When one is deaf and has no oral speech, sign language is a godsend. With it the deaf can acquire a concept of language, a means of communicating, and breaking out of the prison of silence. The metaphor is far more powerful than it might first appear. Sign language is a language in its own right. It is not just a representation of English. It has a different structure from English and the symbols used represent concept rather than English words.[24] So is it with illness. The signs and symptoms of disease stand for concepts of illness, but are not exact representations of the metaphysical language one would need to use if one wanted to convey the same ideas. In our efforts at curing the disease, we use the same means of communication that the patient uses. Our efforts at curing are the sign language that convey our desire to heal. By our willingness to listen to the language of the person who is ill, we listen to the concepts conveyed in the message. But the language, like the language of the deaf, is so limited that our messages will always be inadequate, and we must always decide what the patient's messages really mean.

Atonement

It is our responsibility to interpret this language. We are to make choices, we are to respond, and we are to exercise "our responsible self." [25]

Our acknowledgment of our sin, magnified by our unfulfillable promises and reduced by our willingly shouldering the burdens of the patients, will change our view of God. Each time we try to help a patient, it is God who makes it possible for us to continue helping. We can atone for our failings, and we can be assured that God will forgive us. All of a sudden the interaction between the physician and God becomes different. The physician no longer battles God the enemy in the patient, but rather feels help from God the friend. Whenever we exercise our free choice in helping patients, God is there and He supports us when we are down and crushed. He died and arose from the dead for us. Just so do we make decisions for our patients, acting *in loco Jesu*. And, being more human than he, we must enact our role over and over again in each encounter.

When we try to philosophize about our overburdened humanity we fall into the language of Niebuhr, ponderous, no matter how profound an insight he proclaimed.[25] Saint Paul said it much more concisely:

> … I believe nothing can happen that will outweigh the supreme advantage of knowing Christ Jesus my Lord. For him I have accepted the loss of everything, and I look on everything as so much rubbish if I can have Christ and be given a place in him. I am no longer trying for perfection by my own efforts, the perfection that comes from the law, but I want only the perfection that comes through faith in Christ, and is from God and based on faith. All I want is to know Christ and the power of his resurrection and to share his suffering by reproducing the pattern of his death.[26]

To answer the calling of a physician and to become a mature adult with generativity and integrity, caring and wise, means to do just that: "to share his sufferings by reproducing the pattern of his death," not just once, but over and over again.

But the repeated presence of God and the repeated experience of being forgiven makes sharing his suffering an incredible joyous experience. There is nothing inherently painful in sacrifice – rather the contrary. Taking the role a physician is called to take is a privilege. Being the healer and the living embodiment of Christ's humanity is a joy. We feel the urge to have the best skills in order not to put our calling to shame. We feel strength in our humanity, precisely because we are imperfect in our humanity. Our imperfection allows us to savor God's grace. As physicians we are special because we are forced to partake from that grace more frequently.

When the master, God, said, "Well done thou good and faithful servant," there must have been a smile on the face of the servant. It is joyous to do a job well. There is satisfaction in praise. But nothing is more destructive than praise received and not earned. The joy of being a physician is our reward when we realize our calling, our rebellion, our guilt, and especially our atonement.

EPILOGUE

Epilogue

he exhortation of Saint Paul to the Philippians leaves little room for doubt, little room for avoiding full commitment. Yet doubt remains. If Christ could not face crucifixion once, how can we, being mere humans, face that fate at each patient encounter? Saint Paul confesses his humanity also, when he continues to the Philippians:

> It is not to be thought that I have already achieved all this. I have not yet reached perfection but I press on, hoping to take hold of that for which Christ once took hold of me. My friends, I do not reckon myself to have got hold of it yet.[1]

We must remember, again, that certainty is a very poor substitute for hope. We, too, will falter, we will rise up again and try again, finding ourselves doing wrong one time and truly healing another. Yet, we must proceed.

Some years ago a postdoctoral fellow joined my laboratory staff while I was teaching biochemistry at Vanderbilt University School of Medicine. He was from Israel and an ardent Zionist. I tried to locate an apartment for him before he arrived, and I found the best mix of cost and comfort in the student housing at Scarritt College for Christian Education.[2] Menachem, the fellow, became extremely interested in the phenomenon of Christianity. He found his neighbors in the housing untrained to meet his querying challenge. He therefore asked me what I could recommend if he had to read one book on Christianity other than the Bible. He asked the same from his father-in-law in Israel. Both of us recommended independently Thomas à

The Least Among Thee

Kempis' *The Imitation of Christ*. He read it carefully, and was impressed, but he was bothered by the lack of outward signs of our professed convictions in the students and me. That is, of course, not a new observation, but this time it was made in an acute setting by an honest, searching man, and therefore made a lasting impression on me.

We hardly ever succeed in our imitation of Christ, but we should try and hope that each new attempt will be a little bit better. Our driving force, love for our patients, will make that possible. Thomas à Kempis said, "Vera Magnum est, qui magnam habet caritatem (he is truly great who is great in love).[3]

We can hope for greatness if we can strive for love. We can hope for forgiveness if we use our freedom and select our possibilities in the name of the Lord. There is hope for all when greatness is attainable even by the weak. The weakness of Saint Therese of Lisieux was in fact her power. She knew her inability to be perfect very well:

> I am, I confess, far from practicing what I know I should, yet the mere desire I have to do so gives me peace.[4]

Physicians can have that peace. When they hear their calling and respond, they will meet God as their friend and they will heal with the skill of their profession by their faith. The result will be the joy of service.

NOTES:

Biblical quotes are abbreviated as follows: KJV = King James Version; NEB = New English Bible; RSV = Revised Standard Version; JB = Jerusalem Bible.

Preface:

1. Robert Frost, "Desert Places," in: *The Poetry of Robert Frost*, Lathem EC, editor. New York: Holt, Rinehart & Winston, 1960, p. 296, lines 7-8.

Introduction:

1. The Castle was built in 1890 as a private estate. It was bought in 1893 to become a prep school. However, the Castle and the adjacent area soon became a summer resort. Parents started building cottages and the owners closed the school to create Castle Park, a summer colony. The Castle was operated as the Castle Club and was available for visitors and for retreats. It changed hands again in 1917 and Castle Park flourished under its new owner. However, in 1985 the Castle closed to the general public.
2. Lewis Thomas, "My Magical Metronome," in: Thomas L, *Late Night Thoughts on Listening to Mahler's Ninth Symphony*. New York: The Viking Press, 1983, pp. 45-48.

Chapter I:

1. The meaning of health and disease is an important backdrop against which physician-patient interactions must be understood. A good general resource is: Kenneth L. Vaux, *This Mortal Coil*, San Francisco: Harper & Row, 1978. Ken Vaux and I are friends. We have had regular discussions about the ethics of being a physician.
2. Helmuth M. Thielicke, *I Believe: The Christian's Creed*, Doberstein JW, Anderson HG, translators. Philadelphia: Fortress Press, 1968, pp. xii-xiii.
3. Karl K. Barth, *Credo*, McAfee Brown R, translator. New York: Charles Scribner & Sons, 1962, p. 39.
4. Part of what follows has been published previously, as: J. van Eys, "Lore and Science: Resolving the Dilemma," *The Cancer Bulletin*, 32 (1), 31-36, 1980. That material was presented as part of the Fourth Annual Mental Health Conference of the Department of Pediatrics, The University of Texas MD Anderson Cancer Center, Houston, TX.
5. John L. Dusseau, "The Great Cham as Medical Biographer," *The Pharos*, 42: 10-17, 1979. Dusseau quotes from: H.W. Haggard, "Treatment of King Charles," in: S. Rappaport and H. Wright, editors, *Great Adventures in Medicine*. New York: Dial Press, 1952.
6. Ronald M. Deutsch, *The New Nuts Among the Berries*. Palo Alto, CA: Bull Publishing Company, 1977.
7. Laurie Garrett, *The Coming Plague: Newly Emerging Diseases in a World Out of Balance*. New York: Farrar, Straus, Giroux, 1994.
8. While I was head of the Division of Pediatrics at the University of Texas MD Anderson Cancer Center, we actively participated in that debate. Cf., Jan van Eys, editor, *Research on Children: Medical Imperatives, Ethical Quandaries, and Legal Constraints*. Baltimore, MD: University Park Press, 1978. See also: Paul Ramsey, "Response III, Jan van Eys,: in: Kenneth L. Vaux, Sara Vaux, and Mark Stenberg, *Covenants of Life; Contemporary Medical Ethics in Light of the Thought of Paul Ramsey*, Boston: Kluwer Academic Publishers Philosophy and Medicine, 2002. Volume 77, pp. 211-215.

9. In order to prevent and curtail excesses in research, such as happened in Nazi Germany, laws have been enacted in the United States wherein the federal government mandated that all research, funded by the Government, be reviewed and approved by an independent committee of medical scientists, persons charged with medical care, and lay people. Such committees are called Institutional Review Boards.
10. The quotation is from a translation of the remarkable book, *Klare Wijn; Rekenschap over Geschiedenis, Geheim en Gezag van de Bijbel* ('s Gravenhage: Boekencentrum B.V., 1977). This book was the product of a special commission for the General Synod of the Dutch Reformed Church under the leadership of Professor Dr. L. de Groot and was accepted by the Synod in 1966. The translation cited is by A. Mackie and is published as *The Bible Speaks Again* (Minneapolis, MN: Augsburg Publishing House, 1972.) The original Dutch is somewhat more stilted: "De kerk of prediker of bijbellezer zal alleen dan het gezag van de Schrift, het klemmende appel van het Evangelie – dat ook oordeel en gericht kan zijn – werkelijk doen leven en voelbaar kunnen maken, wanneer hij niet tegenover, maar naast de moderne mens wil staan." (p. 243)

Chapter II:

1. Sir William Osler, "The Reserves of Life," in: McGovern JP, Roland CG, editors, *The Collected Essays of Sir William Osler, Volume II: The Educational Essays.* Birmingham, AL: The Classics of Medicine Library, 1985, pp. 323-332; p. 330.
2. Paul Ramsey, *The Patient as Person: Explorations in Medical Ethics.* New Haven, CT: Yale University Press, 1970.
3. Steve Levenson, The Search for a Philosophy of Medicine, *The Pharos*, 41(1): 2-8, 1979. There will be several references to articles in *The Pharos*, which is the journal of Alpha Omega Alpha (AOA), the medical honor society. That journal represents thinking of those physicians deemed to have been the most promising as students among their peers and

teachers. In the spirit of full disclosure: at the time of writing this book, I was an associate editor of *The Pharos*.

4. Edmund D. Pellegrino and David C. Thomasma, *A Philosophical Basis of Medical Practice; Toward a Philosophy and Ethic of the Healing Professions*. New York: Oxford University Press, 1981, p. 147.

5. Stanley J. Hauerwas, Authority and the Profession of Medicine. This was an unpublished manuscript, which Dr. Hauerwas gave me during one of his visits to Houston in July, 1981. A later version of this paper was published as: Stanley M. Hauerwas, "Authority and the Profession of Medicine," in: G.J. Adich, *Responsibility in Health Care*, Volume 12, Philosophy and Medicine. Boston: Springer, 1982, pp. 83-104.

6. Pellegrino and Thomasma, 1981, p. 148.

7. Edmund D. Pellegrino and David C. Thomasma, *The Virtues in Medical Practice*. New York: Oxford University Press, 1993.

8. Pellegrino and Thomasma, 1981. p. 64.

9. E.R. Babbie, *Science and Morality in Medicine*. Berkeley, CA: University of California Press, 1970. Babbie states, "The patient-physician relation, like any other social relationship, reflects the general values of human morality in a given society" (p. 12).

10. From that realization we began a series of annual conferences that we called "Mental Health Conferences," in which we examined the total care of the child with cancer, alternating a discussion from the perspective of the child and family one year with an examination of a specific profession in the care givers team the next.

11. Jan van Eys, "What do we mean by 'The Truly Cured Child'?" in: Van Eys J, editor, *The Truly Cured Child: The New Challenge in Pediatric Cancer Care*. Baltimore, MD: 1977, pp. 81-98.

12. The analogy is a very strong one. Surgeons are in the forefront of nutrition research, including the free and ready use of hyper-alimentation. The Society for Enteral and Parenteral Nutrition (ASPEN) was started by surgeons.

13. Jan van Eys, "The Truly Cured Child: The Realistic and Necessary Goal in Pediatric Oncology," in: Spinetta J, Deasy-Spinetta P, *Living with Childhood Cancer*. St. Louis, MO: C.V. Mosby Co., 1981, pp. 30-40.

Notes

The statement here was the original text as delivered at the meeting. The published text, in an edited form, appeared on page 38.

14. Jan van Eys, "Is All Well with the Young Man Absalom?" in: Dowell Jr. RE, Copeland DR, van Eys J, editors, *The Child with Cancer in the Community*. Springfield, IL: Charles C Thomas, 1988, pp. 111-117.

15. Jan van Eys, 1977, p. 87.

16. See, for instance, David Callahan, The WHO Definition of Health, The Hastings Center Studies, 1: 13-77, 1973. The original definition was: "The Declaration of Geneva, adopted by the Third General Assembly of the World Medical Association, Geneva, Switzerland, 1948."

17. The concepts of health care delivery in the setting of chronic disease were elaborated in our Sixth Annual Mental Health Conference. See: Jan van Eys, "Health Care Delivery, the Next Step Beyond Cure," in: Becky Pack, Donna R. Copeland, Jan van Eys, editors, *The Nurse Challenged; Person and Professional*. Houston, TX: The University of Texas MD Anderson Hospital and Tumor Institute, 1988.

18. Jan van Eys, 1988, "Health Care Delivery," pp. 3-4.

19. Regular exercise can indeed postpone cardiac deterioration.

20. "The Worried Well" is a widely accepted term that is applied to those persons who are at low risk for a given disease and who do not have that disease, but who nevertheless seek medical attention because they worry that they do have the disease or will have it in the near future. It is widely recognized in the AIDS/HIV community, but is seen in every health-care setting.

21. James L.M. Ferrara, "Medical Students: Future Physicians or Organic Mechanisms?", *The Pharos* 39(2): 62, 1976.

22. Cut-throat Pre-Meds. *Time*, May 20, 1974, p.62.

23. Joseph Garland, "Foreword," in: Joseph Garland, editor, *The Physician and His Practice, Boston: Little Brown and Company*, 1954, p.xi. The gender specific title would not be acceptable today.

24. William A. Tisdale, "On Clinical Caring," *The Pharos* 42 (4): 23-26., 1979.

25. G. L. Engel, "Too Little Science: The Paradox in Modern Medicine." *The Pharos*: 39: 127 –131, 1976.

26. Peter McL. Black, "Must Physicians Treat the 'Whole Man' for Proper Medical Care?" *The Pharos* 39, 8-11, 1976.
27. William A. Tisdale, p.25
28. Gustavo Gutierrez, *A Theology of Liberation. History, Politics, and Salvation.* C. Inda and J. Eagleson, transl. Maryknoll, NY: Orbis Books, 1973, p. 198.
29. What follows is a paraphrase from the text of the closing comments during our Sixth Annual Mental Health Conference, published as Jan van Eys, "To be a Person and to have a Ken,", in Becky Pack, Donna R. Copeland, Jan van Eys, editors, *The Nurse Challenged; Person and Professional.* Houston, TX: The University of Texas MD Anderson Hospital and Tumor Institute, 1988.
30. Robert Massie and Suzanne Massie, *Journey*, New York: Albert E. Knopf, 1975. This is the story of a gifted boy from talented parents. The boy had severe hemophilia.
31. Julian L. Byrd, Ministry to the Dying Patient through Availability, *The Cancer Bulletin*: 26, 115-118., 1974.
32. Erik H. Erikson, *Childhood and Society,* 2nd ed, New York: 1963, W.W. Norton & Co., 1963.
33. Stephen R. Grauber, "Preface." In: E. H. Erikson, Editor, *Adulthood.* New York: W.W. Norton & Co., 1976, pp. vii-xii.
34. Jan van Eys, *Humanity and Personhood.* Springfield, IL:Charles C Thomas, 1981.
35. What follows here is paraphrased from an address given October 9, 1981, during a Biomedical Ethics Symposium, sponsored by the Synod of the Covenant, United Presbyterian Church of the USA and the C.S. Mott Center for Human Growth and Development, Wayne State University, Detroit, MI., entitled, "The Beginning and the End of Life; Creating the Future." My presentation was later published as: Jan van Eys, "Who Then Is normal?" *Church and Society,* 72 (1): 8-16., 1982
36. Jürgen Moltmann, *Experiences of God,* M. Kohl, transl. Philadelphia: Fortress Press., 1980. Moltmann contrasts Kierkegaard and Bloch: "How can we hope if we did not simultaneously fear?" and "One needs

a greater hope if one is not to be numbed by anxiety or totally engulfed by it." (p. 41).

37. Søren Kierkegaard, *Works of Love*, M. Ong and E. Ong, transl. New York: Harper Torchbook Editions, Harper and Row, Publisher, 1964, p. 92.
38. St. Luke, 17:11-19, (KJV)
39. That concept ought to be elaborated far more than is possible here. See: Jan van Eys, "The Normally Sick Child," in: Jan van Eys, Editor, *The Normally Sick Child,* Baltimore, MD: University Park Press, 1979, pp. 9-27.
40. St. Matthew 9:2-8, (NEB).
41. David E. Rogers, "The Doctor Himself Must Become the Treatment." *The Pharos,* 37: 126, 1974. David Rogers was president of the Robert Wood Johnson Foundation, an organization dedicated to the equitable distribution of medical care. He was formerly dean of The Johns Hopkins School of Medicine and before that chairman of medicine at Vanderbilt University School of Medicine. Rogers states that he borrowed the phrase from W. McDermott, "Medicine in Modern Society," in: *Cecil-Loeb Textbook of Medicine,* 13th edition, P. B. Beason and W. McDermott, editors. Philadelphia: W.B. Saunders, 1971.
42. Søren Kierkegaard, 1972, p. 72.

Chapter III:

1. Catalog of the Medical School, the University of Texas Health Science Center at Houston, 1976-1977, p. 2.
2. Ibid., pp. 2,3.
3. Ibid., p. 2.
4. These lines are slightly altered from a short introduction given during a panel discussion on the future at a Biomedical Ethics Symposium, "The Beginning and End of Life; Creating the Future," sponsored by the Synod of the Covenant, United Presbyterian Church of the USA, and the C.S. Mott Center for Human Growth and Development, Wayne State University, Detroit, Michigan, October 9 and 10, 1981.

It was published in: Jan van Eys, "Genetic Medicine; An Axiomatic Afterthought," *Church and Society*, 73: 96-99, 1973.

5. The dominance of psychoanalytic thought is well described by Theodore Isaac Rubin in his diary, published as *Shrink*, New York, NY: Popular Library, 1974. The child psychiatrist Robert Coles gives an interesting meditation on that thinking, in: *The Secular Mind*. Princeton, NJ: Princeton University Press, 1999.

6. The history of pellagra is excellently described in: Elizabeth. W. Etheridge: *The Butterfly Caste: A Social History of Pellagra in the South*. Westport, CT: Greenwood Publishing Company, 1972. See also: Murray Wiener and Jan van Eys, *Nicotinic Acid: Drug, Nutrient, Cofactor*. New York: Marcel Dekker, 1983.

7. There is the real proviso that antibiotics, which used to be so effective against so many infectious diseases, are now often meeting bacterial resistance. Our powerful tools have been blunted by overuse, but we continue to feel confident that new tools can be found.

8. This concept is beautifully discussed by Susan Sontag, in her book *Illness as Metaphor*, New York: Vintage Books, 1979. Cancer has now acquired the same myths, and they are indeed myths. In childhood cancer the disease is no longer incurable, a scourge, or invincible. As early as 1979 we could talk about the curability of cancer: Jan van Eys, and Margaret P. Sullivan, editors, "The Status of Curability of Childhood Cancer," *Proceedings of the 24th Annual Clinical Conference, M.D. Anderson Hospital, Houston, Texas, 1979*, New York: NY: Raven Press, 1980

9. J. F. Fries, "Aging, Natural Death, and the Compression of Morbidity," *New England Journal of Medicine*, 303: 130-135, 1980.

10. J. Peele, Reductionism in the Psychology of the Eighties. Can Biochemistry Eliminate Addiction, Mental Illness and Pain? *American Psychologist*, 36: 807, 1981.

11. Ibid.

12. Thomas Szasz, *The Myth of Mental Illness* (revised edition), New York,: Harper and Row, 1974. See also: Thomas Szasz, *The Theology of Medicine*, New York: Harper and Row, 1977.

Notes

13. Kenneth L. Vaux, *This Mortal Coil, The Meaning of Health and Disease*. San Francisco: Harper and Row, 1978.
14. Albert Camus, *The Plague* (S. Gilbert, transl.) New York: Vintage Books, 1972.
15. Kenneth L. Vaux, "The Child is the Message," in: Jan van Eys, editor, *The Normally Sick Child*. Baltimore, MD: University Park Press, 1989, p. 183.
16. Stanley M. Hauerwas, "Authority and the Profession of Medicine," unpublished essay. A later version was published as Stanley M. Hauerwas, "Authority and the Profession of Medicine," in: G.J. Adich, *Responsibility in Health Care*, volume 12, Philosophy and Medicine. Boston: Springer, 1982, pp. 83-104.
17. Vaux, 1978, p. 183.
18. Pierre Teilhard de Chardin, *Letters to Two Friends,* New York: New American Library, 1968, pp. 75-79.
19. R.L. Stevens, "A President's Assassination," *JAMA*, 246:1674, 1981.
20. Ibid.
21. Ibid.
22. Emil J. Freireich, "Death with Dignity?" *The Cancer Bulletin*, 26: 110-114, 1974.
23. Albert D. Anderson, "Therapeutic Thrust: The Magic in Medicine." *Man and Medicine*, 3: 119-126, 1978.
24. The National Commission for the Protection of Human Subjects of Biomedical and Behavioral Research, *Report and Recommendations for Institutional Review Boards*. Washington, DC: Department of Health, Education, and Welfare, DC, 1978. Publication no.: (OS) 78-0008, p.1.
25. Kenneth L. Vaux, *Morality for the New Medicine,* San Francisco: Harper and Row, 1976, pp. 53-54.
26. Ibid.
27. Jan van Eys, "Should Doctors Play God?" *Perspectives in Biology and Medicine,* 25: 481-485, 1982.
28. Mrs. Billy Graham, "Foreword," in: Claude A. Frazier, ed., *Should Doctors Play God?* Nashville, TN: Broadman, 1971, p. vii.
29. Virginia M. Axline, *Play Therapy* (revised edition), New York: Ballentine Books, 1969, p. 9.

30. Ibid. The gender-specific description is hers.
31. Job 1:21 (NEB)
32. Ibid. 42:2-6
33. *The Complete Poems of Emily Dickinson,* Thomas H. Johnson, editor, Boston: Little, Brown & Company, 1960, p. 619.
34. Genesis 32:26 (NEB)
35. Ibid. 32:31
36. My loose translation of "Nec lussise pudet, sed non incidere ludum."
37. Shakespeare, *Hamlet*, III, 1, 57-60.
38. Bruno Bettelheim, *The Uses of Enchantment, The Meaning and Importance of Fairy Tales.* New York: Vintage Books, 1977, p. 18.
39. *Hamlet,* III, 1, 84-85.
40. The adjective "narcissistic" in this context is deliberate. Cf. Roger J. Bulger, "Narcissus, Pogo, and Lew Thomas Wager," annual oration of the Society for Health and Human Values, Washington, DC, delivered October 26, 1980, and published privately by the society.
41. Erik H. Erikson, *Childhood and Society*, 2nd edition, New York: W.W. Norton and Company, 1963.
42. Richard J. Evans, *Dialogue with Erik Erikson*, New York: E.P. Dutton and Company, 1969, p. 53.
43. Erik Erikson, "Reflections on Dr. Borg's Life Cycle," in: Erik H. Erikson, editor, *Adulthood.* New York: W.W. Norton & Company, 1976, pp. 1-31. It is interesting that Erikson changed his stance between *Childhood and Society* and this article, in calling the antimonies of adulthood generativity versus self absorption, instead of the original generativity versus stagnation. Both are apt but self absorption fits the case of the physician far better.
44. Cary E. Sullivan, "Invocation," *The Pharos,* 44 (3): 23, 1981.
45. Søren Kierkegaard, *Fear and Trembling*, W. Lowrie, transl. Princeton, NJ: Princeton University Press, 1968.
46. William G. Bartholome, "The Shadow of Childhood Cancer and Society's Responsibilities," in: *National Conference on the Care of the Child with Cancer.* New York: The American Cancer Society, 1979, p.165.
47. Ibid. p. 169.
48. Psalm 19:11-14 (NEB).

Notes

Chapter IV:

1. Henry J. Nouwen, *The Wounded Healer,* Garden City, N.Y: 1979, pp. 71-72.
2. Ibid., p. 71. The original passage reads, "If there is any posture that disturbs a suffering man or woman, it is aloofness. The tragedy of Christian ministry is that many who are in great need, many who seek an attentive ear, a word of support, a forgiving embrace, a firm hand, a tender smile, or even a stuttering confession of inability to do more, often find their ministers distant men who do not want to burn their fingers. They are unable or unwilling to express their feelings of affection, anger, hostility or sympathy."
3. John P. McGovern, "Medallions in Medical History: William Osler (1849-1919)." *Harris County Physician,* 17: 27, 1976. Dr. McGovern cofounded the American Osler Society in 1968.
4. Ibid. From that same article the biographical data can be learned: "Osler was born on July 12, 1849, in Bond Head, Ontario, the ninth child of English parents who came to Canada to engage in missionary work. He received his medical degree from McGill University in 1872 and, after two years visiting medical centers in Europe, returned to Montreal to establish his clinical practice. Within a short time he was invited to join the medical faculty at McGill where he quickly established a reputation as an astute clinician and effective young teacher. In 1884, Osler was called to the United States as Professor of Medicine at the University of Pennsylvania. In 1888 he moved to Baltimore, having been chosen the first Chief of Medicine at the new Johns Hopkins Hospital and key organizer of the new medical school as one of the famed 'Hopkins Four,' which included Welch, Halstead, and Kelly. Osler ended his illustrious career in medicine at Oxford as Regius Professor of Medicine from 1905 until his death on December 29, 1919, at the age of 70."
5. Ibid.
6. Rudolph Bultmann was a theologian, best known for his quest for the "Historical Jesus." Cf.: Rudolph Bultmann and five critics, *Kerygma*

and Myth, H.W. Bartch, editor. New York: Harper and Row, 1961. See also: Rudolph Bultmann, *Jesus Christ and Mythology*, New York: Charles Scribners Sons, 1958.

7. William Osler, *A Way of Life*, Springfield, IL: Charles C Thomas, 1969. That particular volume, from which I quote here, was published in commemoration of the fiftieth anniversary of Osler's death.

8. Ibid.

9. John P. McGovern, "Foreword," in: William Osler, *A Way of Life*, Springfield, IL: Charles C Thomas, 1969, p. v-vi.

10. John P. McGovern and Wilburt C. Davison, "Osler and Children," *JAMA*, 210: 2241-2244, 1969.

11. H.K. Faber and R. McIntosh, *History of the American Pediatric Society*, New York: McGraw Hill, 1966, p.12.

12. Osler, 1969, p.12.

13. Francis S. Collins, moderator, Robert L. Ney, Nortin M. Hadler, Campbell W. McMillan, and Charles Mangano, panel members: "The Medical Dilemma: Professional Demands and Personal Needs – A Panel Discussion." *The Pharos*, 41 (2):34, 1978. The quoted remarks were by Dr. Mangano.

14. I have discussed this theme several times before. What follows is an edited version of a previously published article: Jan van Eys, "Why Be an Oncologist?" *Archives of the Founation of Thanatology*, 6: 23, 1977. Another version of the same theme can be found as: Jan van Eys, "Being an Oncologist," *Cancer Bulletin*, 29: 99-103, 1977, and in: Jan van Eys, *Humanity and Personhood*, Springfield, IL: Charles C Thomas, 1981.

15. This assertion is still true, even almost three decades after the original workshop. Much has been learned about cancer biology, targeting chemotherapy to the patient's unique molecular biological makeup, and counteracting side effects. For some cancers, especially childhood cancers and breast cancer, continuous complete, unmaintained remissions have markedly increased. But overall true cures are still not the rule.

16. Margaret Buchhorn, "A Community in Conversation," in: Jan van Eys, ed. *The Truly Cured Child: The New Challenge in Pediatric Cancer Care.* Baltimore, MD: University Park Press, 1977, pp. 123-131.

Notes

17. William G. Bartholome, "The Shadow of Childhood Cancer and Society's Responsibilities," in: *National Conference on the Care of the Child with Cancer.* New York: The American Cancer Society, 1979, p.165.
18. This perception is made clearer when one contrasts death from cancer and from a heart attack. Cancer death is the paradigm for all that is ontologically frightening. This has been discussed elsewhere: Jan van Eys, "To Die from Cancer or from a Heart Attack," in: James Reiffel, Robert DeBellis, Lester C. Mark, Austin H. Kutscher, Paul R. Patterson, and Bernard Schoenberg, editors, *Psychological Aspects of Vascular Diseases.* New York: Columbia University Press, 1980, pp. 204-208. This article appeared previously in *Archives of Tanatology,* 6: 63, 1976.
19. Emil J. Freireich, "Death with Dignity?" *The Cancer Bulletin,* 26: 110-114, 1974.
20. Ibid.
21. John Dewy, *Essays in Experimental Logic,* New York: Dover Publications, 2004.
22. Noam Chomsky, *Reflections on Language,* New York: Pantheon Publications, Inc., 1978.
23. Emil J. Freireich, "Medical Perspective," in: D.G. McCarthy, Ed. *Responsible Stewardship of Human Life.* Saint Louis, MO: The Catholic Hospital Association, 1976, pp.80.
24. Ibid. p. 62.
25. Jan van Eys, "What Do We Mean by the Truly Cured Child?" in: Jan van Eys, editor. *The Truly Cured Child: The New Challenge in Pediatric Cancer Care.* Baltimore, MD: University Park Press, 1977, pp. 81-98.
26. H. Brody, "Hope," *JAMA* 246: 1411-1412, 1981.
27. *The Complete Poems of Emily Dickinson,* Thomas H. Johnson, editor. Boston: Little, Brown & Company, 1960, p. 202.
28. H. Lipkin, "On Lying to Patients," *Newsweek,* June 4, 1979, p. 13.
29. Norman Cousins, "A Layman Looks at Truth Telling in Medicine." *JAMA,* 244: 1929-1930, 1980.
30. Brody, 1981, p. 1411.
31. Psalm 39:7 (RSV).

32. A. Worcester, *The Care of the Aged, the Dying, and the Dead*, Springfield, IL: Charles C Thomas, 1940. I found this comment in: W.R. Phillips, "Patients, Pills, and Professionals: The Ethics of Placebo Therapy." *The Pharos*, 44: 21-25, 1981.

33. Norman Cousins, *Anatomy of an Illness*, New York: Bantam Books, 1981.

34. Andre Malraux, *Lazarus*, T. Kilmartin, transl. New York: Holt, Rinehart and Winston, 1974.

35. Cambridge Research Institute, *Trends Affecting the U.S. Health Care System*, Washington, DC, Department of Health, Education and Welfare, Publication no. HRA 76-14503, U.S. Government Printing Office, 1976.

36. Paul C. Bracken, "The Status of Family Practice," in: Donald Berwick, editor, *The Roles of Family Practice, Internal Medicine, Obstetrics and Gynecology, and Pediatrics in Providing Primary Care.* Report on the Seventy-Third Ross Conference on Pediatric Research. Columbus, OH: 1977, pp. 25-29.

37. F. Douglas Scutchfield, "Prometheus and Sisyphus; Medical Mythology." *The Pharos*, 43: 16, 1980.

38. Walter O. Spitzer, "The Intellectual Worthiness of Family Medicine." *The Pharos*, 40 (3): 2-12, 1977.

39. Julian L. Byrd, "Ministry to the Dying Patient through Availability." *The Cancer Bulletin*, 26: 115-118, 1974.

40. Henry J.M. Nouwen, *The Living Reminder; Service and Prayer in Memory of Jesus Christ.* New York: Seabury Press, 1977, p. 19.

41. K. Medina, "Where Can I Go?" Quoted in: Nettie Katab, "The Mental Health Worker – Interpreting a New World," *The Cancer Bulletin*, 32: 16-18, 1980.

42. Jim Kimball, "To Comfort Always," *The Cancer Bulletin*, 32: 11-12, 1980.

43. Psalm 13:1-4 (NEB)

44. Betty Pfefferbaum, "Rational Decisions, Based on Feelings," *The Cancer Bulletin*, 32: 5-7, 1980.

45. *Jesus Christ, Superstar*. Words and music: Tim Rice and Andrew Lloyd Webber, Decca Records.

Notes

46. Psalm 4:1 (NEB)
47. Psalm 130 4:1. Translation "Out of the depth have I called to thee." (NEB)

Chapter V:

1. Robert Frost, "Desert Places," in: *The Poetry of Robert Frost*, E.C. Lathem, editor, New York: Holt, Rinehart and Winston, 1960, p.296.
2. Austin P. Flannery, editor, *The Documents of Vatican II*. New York: Pillar Books, 1975. The quote is from "Call to Holiness," paragraph 40 of *Lumen Gentium: Dogmatic Constitution of the Church*. The biblical passage is from St. Matthew 5:48 (JB)
3. Robert Frost, "Stopping by Woods on a Snowy Evening." The poem was quoted and the exegesis verified from a lecture by A. Tate: "Inner Weather, Robert Frost as Metaphysical Poet," in: *Robert Frost: Lectures on the Centennial of His Birth*, Washington, DC: Library of Congress, Document no. LC1.14:T18, 1975, pp. 57-68.
4. St. Matthew 25:21 (KJV)
5. Henry J.M. Nouwen, *The Living Reminder; Service and Prayer in Memory of Jesus Christ*. New York: Seabury Press, 1977.
6. Thomas Merton, *He Is Risen*. Niles, IL: Argus Communication, 1975
7. Thomas Merton, *New Seeds of Contemplation*. New York: New Directions Publishing Corporation, 1961, p.165.
8. St. Matthew 7:7 (NEB)
9. St. Matthew 7:33 (NEB)
10. This demand for power because of our all-envisioning wisdom has often been described in the literature. A saga of the common man, so misguided, was given to us by Arjen Miedema, *Gesprekken met Gabriel* [Conversations with Gabriel], Baarn, the Netherlands: Bosch en Keuning, 1947. As a young man I felt and acknowledged temptation and I am not sure the book did not encourage it. Miedema presents a powerful juxtaposition of our real lives and our ideals, using as protagonist a common man in the Netherlands shortly after World War

II, living with the memories of all the horrors, and with the broken promises of the liberation from the German occupation. We expected so much more, and quickly. (I am not aware of a translation of Miedema's book into English)

11. Timothy 2:11-13 (NEB)
12. Cf. Psalm 8:6
13. Psalm 13:1-2 (NEB)
14. Psalm 13:5-6 (NEB)
15. Psalm 22:1 (NEB)
16. James 2:14-21 (NEB).
17. Algernon C. Swinburne, *The Garden of Proserpine,* stanza 11. I used the text available at Poetryfoundation.org.
18. Institutional Review Boards (IRB) are committees appointed at institutions where federally supported biomedical or behavioral research is conducted. They are under the supervision of and report to the Office of Human Research Protection (OHRP) of the Department of Health and Human Services. No human research can be performed without local IRB approval.
19. This represents a very small part of a tremendous problem that American Scientific medicine has generated. Cancer clinical trials have become a mode of therapy, largely because the persons (physicians) who perform these experiments are not mature in the sense discussed in the previous chapter. The issues of science are often ignored. These concerns have been discussed by me elsewhere in great detail: "Pediatric Clinical Trials: Time for Renewal." *Cancer Clinical Trials,* 2: 273-275, 1979 [from which the quote is derived]; "Basic Research versus Clinical Research; Where's the Problem?" *The Cancer Bulletin,* 32: 222-226, 1980; "The Human as Experimental Animal: Necessary or Desirable?" in: Jan van Eys, editor, *Research on Children, Medical Imperatives, Ethical Quandaries, and Legal Constraints.* Baltimore, MD: University Park Press, 1978, pp. 39-51; "The Devil's Being God's Best Inspiration: The Boundary Between Research and Care," in: Kenneth L. Vaux, Sara Vaux, and Mark Sternberg, editors. *Covenants of Life: Contemporary Medical Ethics in Light of the Thought of Paul Ramsey.* Boston: Kluwer Academic Publishers, 2002, pp.177-183.

Notes

20. Karl Barth, *Deliverance to the Captives*. San Francisco: Harper and Row, 1978, p.27.
21. Saint John of the Cross, *The Dark Night of the Soul*, K.F. Rinehart, translator and editor, New York: Frederick Ungar Publishing Co., 1957, p.26.
22. Algernon C. Swinburne, "In Sepulcretis," in: *The Complete Works of Algernon Charles Swinburne; Poetical Works*. Vol. 6, E. Gosse and T.J. Wise, editors. New York: Russell and Russell, 1968, p. 30.
23. Karl Rahner, *Meditations on Hope and Love,* New York: Seabury Press, 1977
24. G. Gustafson, D. Pfetzing and E. Zawolkow, *Signing Exact English* (Revised and Enlarged), Silver Spring MD: Modern Sign Press, 1975.
25. H. Reinhold Niebuhr, *The Responsible Self*. San Francisco: Harper and Row, 1978
26. Philippians 3:8-11 (JB).
27. Matthew 25:23 (KJV)

Epilogue:

1. Philippians 3:12-13 (NEB)
2. Scarritt College was originally founded in Kansas City, Missouri. It was established for the purpose of training young women missionaries. In 1924 it moved to Nashville, Tennessee, where it became Scarritt College for Christian Workers, with strong Methodist ties. In 1981 Scarritt College became a graduate school for Christian Educators. However, enrollment dwindled and the college was closed in 1988. The women's division of the United Methodist Church purchased the buildings and grounds and created the Scarritt-Bennett Center, as a non-profit education, retreat, and conference center with a strong commitment to promoting racial equality, cross-cultural understanding, the empowerment of women, and spiritual renewal. (www.scarrittbennett.org)

3. Thomas à Kempis: *De Imitatione Christi,* R. Bouman, editor. Bussum, the Netherlands: Paul Brand, 1914. My father gave me his copy, which was this edition, on my departure for America.
4. Saint Therese of Lisieux, *The Story of a Soul.* Garden City, NJ: Image Books, 1957, p. 120.

ABOUT THE AUTHOR:

Dr. van Eys was born in the Netherlands in 1929. He came to the United States in 1951 to study at Vanderbilt University in Nashville, Tennessee, where he received his PhD in Biochemistry. He did a post-doctoral fellowship at the Johns Hopkins University. Later he received his MD degree from the University of Washington, School of Medicine in Seattle, Washington. He served on the faculty of Vanderbilt rising to the rank of Professor of Biochemistry, and later also to Professor of Pediatrics. During that time he was for a period a Howard Hughes fellow until his efforts became primarily focused on pediatric hematology/oncology.

In 1973 he was recruited by the University of Texas, MD Anderson Cancer Center in Houston, Texas, where he became Head of the Division of Pediatrics and Chairman of the Departments of Pediatrics and Experimental Pediatrics. In 1987 he was invited to become Chairman of Pediatrics at the University of Texas Medical School in Houston. When in 1994 his wife became seriously ill, he retired from the University of Texas, to return to Nashville, where, in retirement, he was appointed Clinical Professor of Pediatrics and Senior Scholar in the Center for Medical and Research Ethics at Vanderbilt. In 2006 he retired again and was appointed Clinical Professor of Pediatrics, Emeritus.

Especially during his sojourn in Houston, Dr. van Eys was deeply involved in medical ethics and in religious matters, especially as member of the Board of the Institute of Religion in the Texas Medical Center. He served many years as chair of that board.

His late wife was active in special education. She became the supervisor of the Oral Deaf Program of the Houston Independent School District. Their son is a Methodist Minister in Nashville and their daughter is a Child and Adolescent Psychiatrist on the faculty of Vanderbilt.